'WHAT DID I DIE OF?'

The Deaths of Parnell, Wilde, Synge,
and Other Literary Pathologies

John Benignus Lyons, born in Mayo in 1922
and educated at Castleknock and University
College Dublin, was a consultant physician and
neurologist until retirement from Sir Patrick
Dun's. Since 1975 he has been professor of the
history of medicine in the RCSI. A member
of Irish PEN, he wrote three novels under the
pseudonym Michael Fitzwilliam before concentrating on biography with works on Joyce
(1973), Gogarty (1979) and Kettle (1983). His
most recent book is a history of Mercer's
Hospital, Dublin. He lives in Dalkey with his
Welsh wife, Muriel, and has three children
and nine grandchildren.

By the same author

The Citizen Surgeon: A Life of Sir Victor Horsley, FRS, FRCS

James Joyce and Medicine

The Enigma of Tom Kettle

Thrust Syphilis Down to Hell and Other Rejoyceana

etc.

'WHAT DID I DIE OF?'

The Deaths of Parnell, Wilde, Synge, and Other Literary Pathologies

J. B. LYONS

THE LILLIPUT PRESS

First published in 1991 by
THE LILLIPUT PRESS LTD
4 Rosemount Terrace, Arbour Hill,
Dublin 7, Ireland

A CIP record for this
book is available from
the British Library

ISBN 0 946640 79 3

The Lilliput Press receives financial assistance from
The Arts Council/An Chomhairle Ealaíon, Ireland

.

Cover by Butler Claffey Design
Set in 11.5 on 12.5 Bembo by
Seton Music Graphics Ltd of Bantry
and printed in Dublin by
Colour Books of Baldoyle

To my wife, Muriel

Contents

Illustrations

Acknowledgments

The score or so of years that have seen the assembling of my chapters allowed me to profit from discussion with many colleagues in the Section of the History of Medicine of the Royal Academy of Medicine in Ireland. I am particularly grateful to C. Breathnach, D. Coakley, Sir P. Froggatt and F.O.C. Meenan. During more recent times my debt to Ms Mary O'Doherty and Ms Gillian Smith for assistance and typing has steadily increased.

Six of my essays have appeared in periodicals or books perhaps not readily available to the general reader; they are republished by permission of the original editors. The Library staffs at the National Library, the Gilbert Library, the libraries of Trinity College, the Royal College of Physicians of Ireland, the Royal College of Surgeons in Ireland, the Royal Dublin Society, the Royal Irish Academy and the British Library have extended their customary helpfulness. Ms Anne Yandle facilitated my study of Malcolm Lowry's papers in the Special Collections Library, University of British Columbia, Vancouver. Mr David J. Hall of Cambridge University Library sent me his bibliography of Helen Waddell. A photocopy of Reginald Turner's letter was supplied by the library of Reading University.

The president of the Old Limerick Society, Mr Kevin Hannan, an authority on the O'Hallorans, supplied a copy of Sir Dudley Bruce Ross's 'Notes on Family History'. The Board of Trinity College has permitted quotation from Edward Hill's fascinating manuscripts and correspondence and from Helen Waddell's correspondence. Mr Vincent Kinane granted access to his unpublished work on the Dublin University Press. Mr A. Kinsella gave me the benefit of his detailed knowledge of events around St Stephen's Green in the Easter Rising. The late Dr Elizabeth Fitzpatrick provided information about John Knott.

Permission to use copyright material is gratefully acknowledged. My thanks are due to Hamish Hamilton for extracts from Richard Ellmann's *Oscar Wilde*; to the Oxford University Press for extracts from *The Collected Letters of John Synge*, vols I and II (ed. Ann Saddlemyer); to Constable & Co. for quotations from Helen Waddell's *Lyrics from the Chinese*, *The Wandering Scholars*, *Peter Abelard*, *The Desert Fathers*, *Poetry in the Dark Ages*. Extracts from Waddell's *More Latin Lyrics* (ed. Dame Felicitas Corrigan) are sanctioned by Gollancz, who also permit quotations from *Helen Waddell, A Biography* by Dame Felicitas Corrigan. The use of extracts from the late Monica Blackett's *The Mark of the Maker* is agreed by Constable.

Penguin Books and the Society of Authors (representing the James Joyce Estate) have permitted quotations from James Joyce's *Ulysses* and *A Portrait of the Artist as a Young Man*. Penguin Books and Peters Fraser & Dunlop, Ltd (representing Malcolm Lowry's executors) have allowed quotations from Malcolm Lowry's *Selected Letters*, *Under the Volcano* and *Ultramarine*; quotations from *Lunar Caustic* and *Selected Poems* respectively are permitted by Jonathan Cape and City Lights (San Francisco) and by Peters Fraser & Dunlop, Ltd. Oliver D. Gogarty SC has allowed the quotation of lines from Oliver St John Gogarty's 'The Hay Hotel'.

John Benignus Lyons MD, FRCPI

Department of the History of Medicine
Royal College of Surgeons in Ireland
123 St Stephen's Green
Dublin 2

Preface

SIR William Osler (the 'ogry Osler' of *Finnegans Wake*[1]), regius professor of medicine at Oxford University, was apt to say that his most important duty was to keep alive Sir James Murray, an elderly lexicographer, pending the completion of his colossal task of editing the *New English Dictionary on Historical Principles*. The seventh volume of that massive work (1909) defined pathography as 'the description of disease'; its second edition (*The Oxford English Dictionary*, 1989) invests the word with a broader meaning to include 'the study of the life and character of an individual or community as influenced by a disease'. It is to be hoped that this sanction will legitimize the endeavours of pathographers, leading to the acceptance of a genre that is becoming increasingly necessary at a time when 'chat shows' are shaping medicine to emerge as something of a DIY art, and all can juggle with differential diagnosis.

'What did I die of?' Parnell asked when his death was rumoured. His actual death, so dramatic and unexpected, has not yet been adequately accounted for by his biographers, but a diagnosis is offered in one of my essays. The late Richard Ellmann seemed singularly determined to attach a notorious stigma to Oscar Wilde when describing his death, although a careful appraisal of the clinical evidence leads, I submit, to a more acceptable if equally tragic diagnosis.

An extended account of John Millington Synge's ill-health is included in the belief that these details increase appreciation of the magnitude of his achievement. *Deirdre of the Sorrows*, like Mozart's *Requiem*, was written in a phase of terminal illness. One should not, however, relate particular phrases to current suffering – phrases redolent of horror such as 'a tale of blood and broken bodies, and the filth of the grave',[2] or, 'death should be a poor, untidy thing, though it's a queen that dies'[3] – death and ageing are universal themes and in his first play, *In the Shadow of the Glen*, when he was unaware that his disease was progressive, he wrote, 'It's lonesome roads she'll be going and hiding herself away till the end will come and they find her stretched like a dead sheep with the frost on her . . .'.[4]

Yet another largely unexplained aspect of pathography is the apparent ease with which major novelists present graphic portraits of ill-health. Is this instinctive or is it sometimes the outcome of vicarious or actual suffering? The careers of James Joyce and Malcolm Lowry could hardly have been more different, but *Ulysses* and *Under the Volcano* are veritable primers on alcoholism, a theme explored in the final essay in this collection.

The idea of creativity enhanced by suffering is romantic and not easy to displace but despite the existence of exceptional instances[5] the reverse would be the general rule. Ill-health usually retards and destroys. The effects of cerebral pathology, indeed, are sometimes too awful to contemplate. Accordingly I have not attempted to describe in detail how, at the summit of her career, Helen Waddell was tripped up by Alzheimer's disease, but have taken her 'Irish dimension' as the focus of my attention. I was introduced to Waddell's *Wandering Scholars* in 1945 by William Doolin FRCSI, and by a happy chance, just a few years ago, I came across the surgeon-editor's own copy of this golden book on a second-hand dealer's shelf. It contained a slim sheaf of his pencilled notes.[6]

Seventy-five years ago, Tom Kettle died at Ginchy. A constitutional nationalist, he deplored the Easter Rising as destructive to his plans. I have been unable either to confirm or to disprove Robert Lynd's statement that 'he fought in the streets of Dublin to suppress it',[7] but Maurice Headlam[8] seems to have erred in giving an account of his being taken prisoner by Countess Markievicz. It was his brother, Laurence J. Kettle, who was detained by the rebels in the College of Surgeons when they stopped him to confiscate his motor for use as a barricade.[9]

Self-advertisement is frowned upon in the medical profession, which explains why John Knott is regrettably a 'forgotten scholar'. Sylvester O'Halloran does have an established place in medical annals but this Limerick surgeon deserves a more prominent place in national cultural history. Sir William Wilde's avocational interests are well recognized but additional information regarding Wilde as a biographer is now presented.

An element of acerbity, not to say eccentricity, adds piquancy to Edward Hill's character yet Milton's Dublin editor was no mere oddity. Robert Bell, a leading critic, spoke of Dr Hill as 'an accomplished scholar whose intimate acquaintance with classical literature gave great weight to his opinions'.[10]

Oliver Goldsmith surely deserves the objective attention that his biographers have generally failed to direct to his academic status. My earliest essay on Goldsmith, published in a medical journal,[11] was actually written with a wider readership in mind. I am now pleased to have an opportunity to present a revised and extended version to the judgment of the common reader, whom Dr Johnson exalted as a person 'uncorrupted by literary prejudices' and untrammelled by the dogmatism of erudition.[12]

NOTES

1. Genial and learned, Osler merited less than anyone the opprobrium of *Finnegans Wake* – 'this ogry Osler will oxmaul us all' (317.16). Born to the manse in Upper Canada, William Osler (1849–1919) graduated in medicine from McGill College, Montreal, 1872. He held chairs in Montreal, Philadelphia and Baltimore, crowning his career in 1904 by accepting an invitation to become regius professor of medicine at Oxford. Joyce's reference to the humane-killer derives from a valedictory address given by Osler at Johns Hopkins University on 22 February 1905, in which he spoke in humorous vein of the uselessness of men of sixty. He mentioned Trollope's *The Fixed Period*, which envisaged a College to which at sixty men retired for a contemplative year before peaceful extinction by chloroform. The audience enjoyed Osler's little joke. Next morning the newspaper headings blazoned his words as a serious message of sinister intent – Osler Recommends Chloroform at Sixty.
2. John M. Synge, *The Complete Plays* (ed. T. R. Henn) (London 1981), p. 245.
3. *Ibid.*, p. 258.
4. *Ibid.*, p. 92.
5. Sir George Pickering argued in *Creative Malady* (London 1974) that by enforcing solitude and leisure, illness may bring advantages to the creative. Certain exceptional individuals such as the late Christy Brown and Davoren Hanna are fulfilled creatively despite extraordinary handicaps.

6. For an account of William Doolin (1887–1962), surgeon to St Vincent's Hospital and editor of the *Irish Journal of Medical Science*, see Introduction to William Doolin's *Dublin's Surgeon-Anatomists and Other Essays* (ed. J. B. Lyons) (Dublin 1987), pp. 13–48.
7. Robert Lynd, *If the Germans Conquered England* (London 1917), p. 139.
8. Maurice Headlam, *Irish Reminiscences* (London 1947), p. 175.
9. Frank Robbins, *Under the Starry Plough* (Dublin 1977), p. 107.
10. Robert Bell, 'John Milton' in *Eminent Literary and Scientific Men*, vol. 1 (London 1839), p. 252.
11. J. B. Lyons, 'The Mystery of Oliver Goldsmith's Medical Degree', *Irish Journal of Medical Science* (1962), 121–41.
12. Virginia Woolf, *The Common Reader* (London 1925), p. 11.

1

Sylvester O'Halloran, 1728–1807*

THE third son of Michael O'Halloran, a substantial Catholic farmer, and his wife, Mary McDonnell, Sylvester O'Halloran was born at Caherdavin, County Clare, on 31 December 1728.[1] Little is known of his childhood and youth. His mother's kinsman, Seán Claragh McDonnell (1691–1754), a man accomplished in Greek, Latin and Irish, the founder of the Court of Poetry of Coshma, was one of his early instructors and he attended a school in Limerick run by the Reverend Robert Cashin, a Protestant clergyman. His schoolmates included Peter Woulfe (1727–1803), the inventor or popularizer of 'Woulfe's bottle', until recently a standard piece of laboratory equipment.[2]

The lack of information about Sylvester O'Halloran's youth challenged the imagination of Ronan Sheehan, whose *Boy with an Injured Eye* is based on O'Halloran's career. Sheehan's interesting but improbable fictional account presents the eleven-year-old boy at Seán Claragh McDonnell's school, his choice of career already made:

'I want to be a physician when I grow up,' Sylvester said [to his teacher, who gives the lad Galen's anatomy to translate]. 'I need hardly tell you of the medical people on your side of the family. Máire has often spoken to me of them. She gets me medical books and pamphlets to read. Also it is a profession in which a Catholic may advance.'[3]

The educational difficulties faced by Catholics in eighteenth-century Ireland were circumvented by the O'Hallorans. At sixteen, the eldest, Joseph Ignatius, went to the Jesuit College in Bordeaux.

* Communication to the annual general meeting of The Eighteenth-Century Ireland Society in 1989; published in *Eighteenth-Century Ireland* (1989), IV, 65–74.

He joined the Society eventually and held chairs successively in rhetoric, philosophy and divinity. The middle brother, George, a jeweller and a man of property, may have been apprenticed locally but Sylvester went abroad to study surgery.

He would have been sixteen or seventeen when he set off to face the ordeal of a sea voyage:

in a passage from Dublin to Chester we met with a most violent storm, and after beating the sea for three days we were at length driven into Milford Haven. Being naturally tender, and lying in a cabin all the time, unable to keep anything on my stomach, my legs became so swelled with cold, that when we were preparing to land, I found myself unable to stand, yet I had no pain. I was carried late into the boat, and from thence to my lodgings, when I begged to lie down; and after an hour's refreshing sleep, awoke, but with exquisite pain.[4]

When his health permitted, he went on to London, where in 1745 he seriously entertained the idea of going north to join Bonnie Prince Charlie. He became acquainted with Richard Mead, a leading physician, of whom Samuel Johnson remarked: 'Dr Mead lives more in the broad sunshine of life than almost any man.'[5] He watched Hillmer and Chevalier Taylor operate and studied their methods closely. Those itinerant eye surgeons attracted sufferers from cataract prepared to face almost any risk to recover their sight.

He may have gone next to Leyden and then to Paris. Early in 1749, O'Halloran returned to Limerick and set up in practice. The city had a population of approximately 30,000 and is described in Young's *Tour of Ireland*:

That city is very finely situated, partly on an Island formed by the Shannon. The main part, called Newtown Pery . . . is well built. The houses are new ones, of brick, large and in right lines. There is a communication with the rest of the town by a handsome bridge of three large arches . . . there are docks, quays, and a custom house which is a good building faces the river, and on the opposite bank is a large quadrangular one, the house of industry. This part of Limerick is a very cheerful place.[6]

A suitable background, then, for an ambitious surgeon. Sylvester O'Halloran dressed the part, wearing an impressive French wig and carrying a gold-headed cane. He was known to be writing a book (an effective advertisement) and must have mystified the populace by ascending the steeple of St Mary's Church with air-filled bladders.[7] The manuscript of *A New Philosophical & Medical*

Treatise on the Air is among the treasures of the Royal Irish Academy, of which O'Halloran became a member about 1787. *A Treatise on the Glaucoma, or Cataract* was published in Dublin in 1750.

O'Halloran married Mary Casey of Ballycasey, County Limerick, in 1752.[8] They had four sons and a daughter and lived at Change-lane, moving later to Merchants' Quay. He was one of the founders of the County Limerick Infirmary, which opened with four beds in 1761 and moved to larger premises in St Francis's Abbey in 1765.

His mind was much occupied by the surgical problems of the day and with the intention of improving current operative methods he performed operations on cadavers. *A New Method of Amputation* appeared in 1763; his book on *Gangrene and Sphacelus* came out in 1765; his most mature surgical work, *A New Treatise on External Injuries of the Head*, was published in 1793. The study on head injuries leaves one in no doubt that O'Halloran was a conservative and reflective surgeon, unwilling to subject patients precipitantly to trepanation, a widely favoured but highly dangerous method of treatment. He had a clear concept of concussion and of compression of the brain by depressed fractures or effusions of blood and pus. Cerebral compression required surgical intervention, which should be avoided in concussion.[9]

The Treatise on Injuries of the Head, ostensibly a surgical monograph, is also a contribution to social history. Violence was commonplace and aggravated by alcohol. 'I have had no less than four fractured skulls to trepan on a May morning,' wrote O'Halloran, 'and frequently one or two.' Fairs, patrons and hurling matches frequently ended in bloodshed:

there is no part of the habitable globe, that for half a century past, has afforded such an ample field for *observations on injuries of the head*, as Ireland in general; this province of Munster in particular! for our people, invincibly brave, notwithstanding the cruel oppressions they have suffered for a century past, and highly irritable, soon catch fire: a slight offence is frequently followed by serious consequences; and sticks, stones, and every other species of offence next to hand, are dealt out with great liberality! To this add the frequent abuse of spirituous liquors, particularly whiskey, which has, unhappily for the *morals* and *constitutions* of the people, found its way to every part of the kingdom![10]

The horse occupied the role as a traumatic agent now taken by motor vehicles. Industrial accidents were important then as now. Gentlemen still resorted to duelling. The causes of 78 cases of head injury reported by O'Halloran (out of more than 1500 cases) may be grouped as follows: personal violence: 43; falls from horses: 15; accidents at work: 7; children kicked by horses: 6; falls: 6; duel: 1.

John Evans, a labourer, fell from a scaffold in November 1767 when the new Custom House was being built. The owner of one of the many sloops that carried turf on the Shannon, 'being in liquor', when going on board from the quay, 'he fell in, head foremost'. Furious encounters were generally between rowdy males but 'William Davitt, clothier of this City, had some dispute with a stout, athletic young wench. . . . He called her by some hard name, and she directly prostrated him. He fell on his back, and she seized a large brass weight, and struck him repeatedly on the left side of the coronal, a little above the frontal sinus.'[11]

The most savage incident reported by O'Halloran followed a seizure of property:

Wm O'Neill, sportsman to the late Colonel Quin, heading a party to take a forcible possession of lands, within four miles of this city, in August 1778, was attacked by the people in opposition and his party routed. He singly stood on his defence, and peremptorily refused to give up his arms. . . . He retreated to a cabin, and swore he would kill the first man that followed him. He presented his piece; it missed fire and he was soon overpowered. Repeated blows could not bring him to the ground. He for some time covered his head with the right fore arm 'till it was fractured, as was also the left, in succeeding to this melancholy office. – He received a very extended wound on the upper part of the left parietal, which laid the bone bare for about two inches. . . .[12]

Apart from his professional work, O'Halloran participated enthusiastically in the life of his city; he was president of the Free Debating Society in 1772 and in 1783 was elected to the Citizens of Limerick Committee set up to enquire into the state of the Shannon navigation. His principal avocation was history and he was the author of *An Introduction to the Study of the Antiquities of Ireland* (1770), *Ierne Defended* (1774)[13] and *A General History of Ireland* (1775). While generally well received, these books were not accorded universal acclaim – one critic advised the doctor to 'drop any more scribbling, and mind the Systole and Diastole of the human body, which I suppose you are better acquainted with than history'.

The preface to Charlotte Brooke's *Reliques of Irish Poetry* (1789) acknowledged her 'Innumerable obligations' to Sylvester O'Halloran, who had made his collection of manuscripts available to her and contributed 'An Introductory Discourse to the Poem of Conlock', which Miss Brooke referred to as 'an ornament and an honour to my work'. She speaks of his 'inestimable' *Introduction to the History & Antiquities of Ireland* (*sic*) as 'a work fraught with learning, rich with the treasures of ages, and animated by the very soul of Patriotism, and of genuine Honor!'[14]

Using a novelist's licence, Ronan Sheehan takes us into the mind of the prolific historiographer who has accepted the duty of refuting British historians who, to justify colonization, have represented the Irish as uncouth and primitive. 'The native tradition [O'Halloran reasoned] needed support because it contained many propositions that were, to say the least, unlikely. To write it down required a special kind of faith, or blindness. Indeed, it required the sacrifice of his reputation as a scholar.'[15] Sheehan's explanation for O'Halloran's inflation of our past glories is kinder but less convincing than a judgment of J. C. Beckett, who placed him more soberly among those sympathizers with the old order who sought 'to vindicate its claims by uncritical admiration for the achievements of pre-Norman Ireland'.[16]

O'Halloran in Miss Brooke's *Reliques* pictures an heroic age enriched by forgotten ideals and virtues: [17]

With us chivalry flourished from the remotest antiquity: there were five orders of it; four for the provinces, and one confined to the blood-royal; and so highly was the profession respected among us, that a Prince could not become a candidate for the monarchy, who has not the Gradh-Gaoisge, or order of Knighthood, conferred upon him. At a very tender age, the intended candidate had a golden chain hung round his neck, and a sword and spear put into his hands. At seven years old he was taken from the care of women, and deeply instructed in Philosophy, History, Poetry and Genealogy. The using his weapons with judgment, elegance and address, was also carefully attended to; principles of Morality were sedulously inculcated, and a reverence and tender respect for the Fair, completed the education of the young hero.[18]

A prolific letter-writer, O'Halloran's correspondents included Edmund Burke and Charles O'Conor of Belangare.[19] Four of his letters to O'Conor are devoted largely to a discussion of Macpherson's verses. He offered his copy of O'Clery's 'Irish Vocabulary

or Seansan Nuad' to O'Conor and wished to borrow from him
an Irish translation of Hippocrates. He advised him about an eye
complaint:

You are pleased to request my Advice on this point, & with the greatest
Cordiality you have it – I do think the head should be all over shaved, and
washed Every morning in cold Water, & the Eyes in soft linnen moistened
with Cold Spring Water, & that often in a day; refrain as much as you can
from close reading or writing, & in some Cases get an Amanuensis – If the Eyes
should be dull & heavy get a small bottle of genuine Spiritus Volatilis Aromaticus.
Drop some on your own, or an Assistant's hands, & after speedily rubbing
them together, apply briskly to the Eyes. This if done right, will Act like Elec-
tricity, brisken the Circulation in the humours, & make them water a little.[20]

Tomás Ó Míocháin, a well-esteemed schoolteacher from
Ennis in County Clare, wrote a poem in O'Halloran's honour:

Do charas féin go feas
seabhac is aoirde mórmheas,
easna cnuais don cheap Chuinn,
ollamh oirdhearc gan eascaoin.

Is caoin 'sas cneasda caom, ionraic,
fionmahr, fleágach, feasach, fíorchlúmhamhuil
an tsaoi ghlic ghasda a reacht na bpríomhúghadar,
craobh de cheap ghlain cheart Uí Alludhráin.[21]

O'Halloran also was featured in Gilborne's doggerel, *The Medical
Review* (1775), a compendium of eighteenth-century medical
worthies.

In Limerick O'Halloran resides
And o'er the County Hospital presides;
Excels in Surgery and healing Arts,
With flowing Pen displays uncommon Parts;
Relates with Ingenuity and Truth
How brave Milesius with his Fleet came o'er,
And chosen Scythians from Hesperia's Shore,
Old Ireland's first Inhabitants subdu'd . . .[22]

Dublin's surgeons and barbers were incorporated on 18 October
1446 as the Fraternity or Guild of St Mary Magdalene, their
emblem the red and white striped pole that until recently indicated the presence of a barber's shop. The link between barbers
and surgeons stems from the rude practice of healing in medieval
monasteries and was increasingly resented by the surgeons whose
art gained in stature with the accumulation of knowledge.

O'Halloran's *Proposals for the Advancement of Surgery in Ireland* (1765), an admirable blueprint, advocated in summary: 'That a decent and convenient edifice be created in the capital, and three professorships founded'; that a register of surgeons be kept; that candidates for recognition must apply for examinations, which should be free of expense; that a printed list should be published annually of the registered surgeons and men-midwives.[23]

Traditionally O'Halloran's *Proposals* is credited with having played a vital part in the foundation of the Royal College of Surgeons in Ireland. This is largely conjectural but supported by the fact that the Dublin Society of Surgeons founded in 1780 elected its provincial colleague to honorary membership. The Royal College of Surgeons in Ireland received its charter on 11 February 1784 and two years later Sylvester O'Halloran was elected an honorary member (equivalent to the present-day fellowship).[24]

His wife's death in 1782 grieved and dispirited him and some years later he alluded to his bereavement in a letter to Edmund Burke.[25] 'I should long since have Ushered into the World a new Edition of my treatise on Gangrene . . . but the immature death of an Amiable and Accomplished wife has for a long time suspended its execution . . .'. The widower survived for a quarter of a century, the loneliness of the house on Merchants' Quay lightened early in the new century by the laughter of his grandchildren.[26]

At least two of Sylvester O'Halloran's grandsons settled in Australia. These were Thomas and William O'Halloran, sons of Sir Joseph O'Halloran (1763–1843), the surgeon's youngest son, who, having given 53 years' uninterrupted service in India, was made an honorary member of the Royal Irish Academy and freeman of the city of Limerick.[27]

Thomas Shuldham O'Halloran (1797–1870) was born at Berhampore, India, but he and his sister, Ellen, were sent to spend their early years in Limerick with their grandfather, who, at his death, left the little girl a gold watch and gave his own silver watch to the boy. The children were moved in 1807 to the care of their mother's family, the Baylys of Redhill, Surrey.

After serving in India, Thomas O'Halloran retired from the army in 1835 and sailed with his family to Australia, settling at a place some miles south of Adelaide near the river Sturt, now known as O'Halloran's Hill. He was appointed commissioner of police, in which office he subdued the Aborigines with the ruthless efficiency the Victorians did not find incompatible with Christianity, in which sphere he was one of the founders of Christ Church, O'Halloran's Hill. He was elected member of the first parliament of South Australia in 1857. A progressive farmer, he cultivated wheat with great success.[28]

William Littlejohn O'Halloran (1806–85), Joseph's ninth child, was born in Ireland. He entered the army at eighteen, purchased a company in 1838 but retired two years later and emigrated to Australia. He became a member of the Audit Board and in 1851 was appointed Auditor General of Western Australia.[29]

Paris, where Sylvester O'Halloran had repaired to in the mid-century, was then the ideal centre for aspirant surgeons and its great hospitals, the Hôtel-Dieu, La Charité, and others, attracted many foreign students. The young Irishman's movements in Paris cannot be traced, other than his attendance at the lectures of Antoine Ferrein in 1747–8, but he was especially impressed by the *Académie Royale de Chirurgie*, which clearly influenced his *Proposals for the Advancement of Surgery in Ireland*:

In France [he wrote] the advancement of surgery has been a particular object of government, for above a century past, besides the different professorships founded, and pensions bestowed on particular men of merit; persons pretending to eminence in any particular brand of the healing art were sure of public countenance. From this attention of the state, surgery began to flourish in a remarkable degree there; and M. Voltaire places the advancement of our profession, as one of the memorable transactions of Lewis XIV.[30]

As the *Académie Royale de Chirurgie* may thus be seen as the model for our surgical college, it is interesting to note that it was largely the creation of Georges Mareschal, whose father, John Marshall, left Ireland with the Wild Geese to settle in France. Mareschal was *premier chirurgien* to Louis XIV and Louis XV and the latter granted him a charter for a *Société Académique* in 1731.[31]

O'Halloran was familiar with the writings of the first members of the French Academy of Surgery, Jean-Louis Petit (1674–1750), François de la Peyronie (1678–1747), and others. He was also widely read in the literature of eye surgery and refers to the French classics, *Traité de la cataracte* by Michel Brisseau and *Les Maladies des yeux* by Charles St Yves in his own treatise. He agreed with them that a cataract is opacification of the lens, he introduced a few anatomical discoveries, and suggested a modification of the current method of 'couching' the cataract.

He did not mention the new operation introduced by Jacques Daviel, extraction of the lens.[32] This was not published until 1752 and Daviel's arrival in Paris coincided with O'Halloran's departure. Before long the latter was performing extractions and considering possible modifications. As Daviel used a needle and scissors to divide the cornea scarring was inevitable. O'Halloran introduced a specially designed, sharply pointed double-edged and slightly convex knife and by making his incision through the sclerotic (white coat of the eye) hoped to avoid the opaque scar in the transparent cornea.[33]

It may be affirmed in conclusion that O'Halloran profited from his stay in Paris, going on to attain national recognition in his profession, but, rather than select any single contribution for which he should be remembered, his real significance may be as a type of cultured, well-informed Catholic gentleman that cannot have been uncommon in his century. His reaction to the revolution in France regrettably is unknown. When writing to Edmund Burke on 15 September 1793, he confined himself to Irish and personal matters[34] but as the century ended he was strongly opposed to the Act of Union. His name – O'Halloran MRIA – appeared in the *Limerick Chronicle* for 15 January 1800 in a list of signatures resisting the proposed Union. And with thirteen other freeholders he requested the sheriffs to convene their bailiwick 'at the nearest convenient day, to consider the propriety of Petitioning Parliament against the Measure of Legislative Union with Great Britain'. His disgust to see his country 'from an *Imperial and Independent State*, reduced to its present situation',[35] impelled him to publish a new edition of *An Introduction to and a History of Ireland* (1803).

Old age advanced relentlessly. The Reverend James Hall, who visited Limerick in 1807, wrote in his *Tour Through Ireland*:

I found Dr O'Halloran the celebrated antiquarian, to whom I had been introduced, old, infirm, and confined to his chair . . . The Doctor who had considered the matter minutely, and has had the best information, is of opinion, that there are above two hundred thousand individuals in the County of Limerick (which is but a small one), yet it could be made, with tolerable cultivation, to support three times that number.[36]

He died in his home at Merchants' Quay during the night of Tuesday, 11 August 1807 and his remains were laid in the family vault in Kileely Cemetery. A memorial tablet was set into the front of the vault by St Senan's Historical Society in 1978. A foot-bridge over the Abbey river is named O'Halloran Bridge and Limerick's recently opened post-graduate medical teaching centre also commemorates the name of Sylvester O'Halloran.

NOTES

1. [W. R. Wilde], 'Illustrious Physicians and Surgeons in Ireland. No. VI. Sylvester O'Halloran, M.R.I.A.', *Dublin Quarterly Journal of Medicine*, V (1848), 223–50; *Dictionary of National Biography*, XIV, pp. 91–2; J. B. Lyons, 'Sylvester O'Halloran', *Irish Journal of Medical Science* (1963), 217–32, 279–88; K. Hannan, 'A Forgotten Limerick Genius', *The Old Limerick Journal*, 22 (1987), 4–7.

2. Woulfe went to Paris on O'Halloran's advice to study under Rouelle. He appears to have been mildly eccentric in his later years, a belated believer in transmutation procedures and given to attaching prayers to his apparatus. He was, nevertheless, a competent and resourceful chemist and described the preparation of ethyl chloride. He was elected to the Royal Society in 1767. See E. L. Scott, 'Peter Woulfe' in C. C. Coulson (ed.), *Dictionary of Scientific Biography* (New York 1980), 14, pp. 508–9.

3. Ronan Sheehan, *Boy with an Injured Eye* (Dingle 1983), p. 27.

4. Sylvester O'Halloran, *A Complete Treatise on Gangrene and Sphacelus* (London 1765), p. 146.

5. F. H. Garrison, *An Introduction to the History of Medicine* (Philadelphia 1929), p. 390.

6. Arthur Young, *A Tour in Ireland* (Dublin 1780), ii, p. 2.

7. J. B. Lyons, 'Sylvester O'Halloran's Treatise on the Air', *Irish Medical Journal*, 76 (1983), 37–9.

8. An entry in Sylvester O'Halloran's diary notes on 16 November 1752 refers to his marriage: 'Married privately, without consulting our parents on either side, Mary Casey, amiable in her person, of the sweetest, and most human disposition possessed of the most exalted principles of Religion, of unbounded charity and benevolence to the whole human race.' Sir Dudley Bruce Ross (b. 1892), whose mother was Thomas Shuldham O'Halloran's granddaughter, Annie Isabella (b. 1863), used the diary when compiling 'Notes on Family History' (unpublished); its present whereabouts is unknown.

9. D. S. Gordon, 'Penetrating Head-Injuries', *Ulster Medical Journal*, 57 (1988), 4–6; J. B. Lyons, 'Irish Contributions to the Study of Head-Injury in the Eighteenth Century', *Irish Journal of Medical Science* (1959), 401–12.

10. Sylvester O'Halloran, *A New Treatise on the Different Disorders Arising from External Injuries of the Head* (Dublin 1793), p. 4.
11. *Ibid.*, p. 328.
12. *Ibid.*, p. 222.
13. This work contains 'A candid refutation of such passages in the Rev. Dr Leland's, and the Rev. Mr Whitaker's work, as seem to affect the authenticity and validity of ancient Irish history.'
14. Charlotte Brooke, *Reliques of Irish Poetry* (Dublin 1789).
15. Ronan Sheehan, *op. cit.*, p. 59.
16. J. C. Beckett in T. W. Moody and W. E. Vaughan (eds), *A New History of Ireland, IV, Eighteenth-Century Ireland* (Oxford 1986), p. lxi.
17. When Bishop Milner of Wolverhampton was given O'Halloran's *Study of the History and Antiquities of Ireland* in 1816, he thanked the donor, saying: 'For my own part, I was glad that I am not obliged to admit, as articles of faith, all the wonderful things contained in this primaeval history . . .'; Brian McDermot (ed.), *The Catholic Question in Ireland and England: The Papers of Denys Scully* (Dublin 1988), p. 600.
18. Sylvester O'Halloran in *Reliques of Irish Poetry*, p. 5.
19. J. B. Lyons (ed.), 'The Letters of Sylvester O'Halloran', *North Munster Antiquarian Journal*, IX (1963), 163–81.
20. *Ibid.*, p. 174.
21. *Eighteenth-Century Ireland*, 1 (1986), 85–9, for the entire poem edited by Diarmuid Ó Muirithe. Relatively little is known of Ó Míocháin but see Brian O'Looney, *A Collection of Poems by the Clare Bards*: 'I do not know when he died but his feeling appeal to the Irish in 1798 was I believe his last poetic composition' (Dublin 1863), p. vi. A poem referring to Washington's victory over Howe at the evacuation of Boston, 17 March 1776, was published by the Colonial Society of Massachusetts: Thomas O'Meehan, *An Eighteenth-Century Irish Song Relating to Washington* (Cambridge, Mass. 1911).
22. John Gilborne, *The Medical Review* (Dublin 1775), p. 47.
23. Sylvester O'Halloran, *Proposals for the Advancement of Surgery in Ireland* (appendix to the *Treatise on Gangrene*, 1765), pp. 287–9.
24. J. D. H. Widdess, *The Royal College of Surgeons in Ireland and its Medical School, 1784–1966*, 2nd ed. (Edinburgh 1967), p. 168.
25. 'Letters', pp. 41–2.
26. Three of his children, Michael, Catherine and Thomas, predeceased him. Michael (b. 1754) married a niece of Lord Fitzgibbon but was killed by a fall from a horse in July 1782, leaving no issue. He is referred to in his father's *diary*: 'Born with great talents, but greatly perverted; he has been a constant source of distress to his amiable mother and to me till his death which was sudden and unexpected.' John O'Halloran, a captain in Colonel Brown's regiment of American Loyalists, was later Secretary to the Governor of the Bahama Islands. His son, Sylvester, died in Jamaica without issue in 1835.
27. *DNB*, XIV, pp. 950–1 and Ross 'Notes': While serving in Bengal in 1780, Joseph O'Halloran was introduced to a young visitor from England,

Frances Bayly, who was staying with the family of Colonel Showers. She was a daughter of Captain Nicholas Bayly, MP for Anglesey and formerly of the Grenadier Guards, and a niece of the Earl of Uxbridge. His courtship was opposed by Colonel Showers, by Miss Bayly's parents and possibly by Sylvester O'Halloran but they married in Calcutta on 1 December 1790. Joseph's description of his bride may have reminded his father of his own enthusiastic diary-entry quoted above. 'To an elegance of figure, and a dignity of manners, Miss Bayly joined a mind exalted by every virtue and excellence which could adorn a woman. I early admitted her personal ease and accomplishment and the superiority of her understanding soon completed the conquest her beauty began.'

28. Kevin Hannan, 'The O'Hallorans in South Australia', *The Old Limerick Journal*, 23 (1988), 30–4.
29. The president of the Old Limerick Society, Mr Kevin Hannan, kindly supplied me with a copy of Sir Dudley Bruce Ross's 'Notes on Family History', which lists other members of Sir Joseph O'Halloran's family – six sons who saw active service: Charles Sylvester 1791–1812, St George James 1799–1815, Henry Dunn 1800–71, Edward 1802–31, Joseph Palmer 1807–25, John Nicholas b. 1810 – and five surviving daughters, who married soldiers: Anne Helen 1795–1856, Sophia Sherburne 1803–32, Jane Baillie b. 1808, Frances Franklin 1812–78, Marie Nugent 1813–48.
30. Sylvester O'Halloran, *Proposals*, p. 271.
31. William Doolin, *Dublin's Surgeon-Anatomists and Other Essays* (ed. J. B. Lyons) (Dublin 1987), pp. 113–33.
32. A. Hubbell, 'Jacques Daviel and the Beginning of the Modern Operation of Extraction of Cataract', *Journal of the American Medical Association*, 39 (1902), 117–85.
33. Sir William Wilde, himself a pioneer in ophthalmic surgery, suggests that O'Halloran made his incision 'at the junction of cornea and sclerotica . . .', *op. cit.*, 236.
34. 'Letters', p. 41.
35. Sylvester O'Halloran, *An Introduction to and a History of Ireland* (Dublin 1803), i, p. iv.
36. J. Hall, *Tour Through Ireland* (London 1813), p. 301.

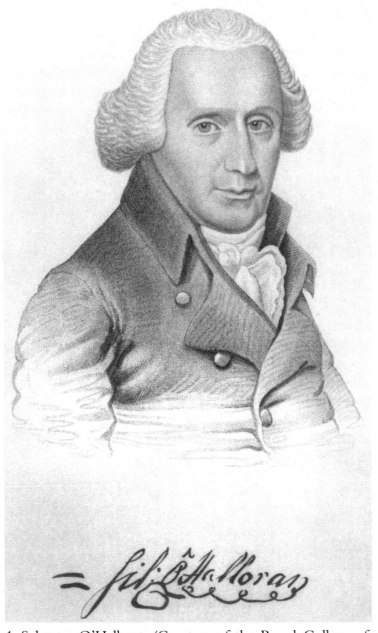

1. Sylvester O'Halloran (Courtesy of the Royal College of Surgeons in Ireland)

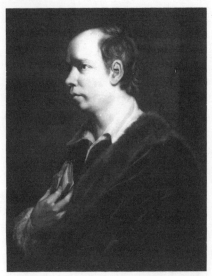

2. Oliver Goldsmith by Sir Joshua Reynolds (Courtesy of the National Gallery of Ireland)

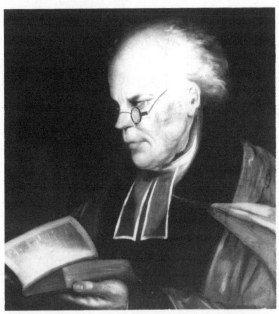

3. Edward Hill MD (Courtesy of the Royal College of Physicians of Ireland)

2

The Vexed Question of Oliver Goldsmith's Medical Degree

OLIVER Goldsmith agreed to dine with the Cradocks[1] in February 1774 on the understanding that he would not be asked to eat anything. He took wine and biscuits but his talk was forced. Towards the end of March an acquisitive visitor to his rooms at Brick Court in the Temple asked if he could take a sheet of paper on which some lines were written. 'In truth you may, my boy,' Dr Goldsmith said, 'for it will be no use to me where I am going.'[2] Since his death on 4 April 1774, a score of biographers and others have disagreed about his medical degree. Most of them convey the impression of having given the matter little thought. Exceptions to this stricture are Sir Ernest Clarke, Sir Raymond Crawfurd and T.P.C. Kirkpatrick, and also Goldsmith's contemporaries. Before giving details of their conclusions I shall outline the Irish poet's unarguable connections with medicine.

When William White Cooper assigned Pallas as the poet's birthplace in his 'Narrative of the Last Illness and Death of Oliver Goldsmith, M.D.' (1848), the editor of the *Dublin Quarterly Journal of Medical Science*, Mr (later Sir) William Wilde, a native of County Roscommon, pointed out that most of Goldsmith's early biographers believed otherwise. 'The late Robert Jones Lloyd, Esq.,[3] has often shewn us the room in which the poet was born, at Ardnagowan (now Smith Hill), near Elphin . . . '.[4] Drs Michael Cox and John Knott and the Rev J.J. Kelly DD, MRIA, have also supported the traditional claim of this locality to be regarded as Goldsmith's birthplace. Father Kelly marshalled the arguments fully in *The Early Haunts of Oliver Goldsmith*.[5]

From those well-loved haunts the lad moved to Dublin and in 1752, urged by his cousin, Isaac Goldsmith, Dean of Cloyne, to study medicine, Oliver Goldsmith BA entered Edinburgh University, where Joseph Black, the discoverer of carbon dioxide, was a fellow student.[6] Goldsmith's signature appears in the *Obligation Book* of the Royal Medical Society under the date 13 January 1753 and his criticism of his teachers was penetrating:

the first and most Deserving Mr Monro[7] Professor of anatomy. This man has brought the science he Teaches to as much perfection as it is capable of and not content with barely Teaching anatomy he launches out into all the branches of Physick where all his remarks are new and useful. . . . Plummer Professor of chemistry understands his business well but delivers himself so ill that he is but little regarded. Alston Professor of Materia Medica speaks much but to little purpose. The Professors of Theory and Practice say nothing but what we may find in the books laid before us and speak that in so droning and heavy a manner that their hearers are not many degrees in a better state than their Patients.[8]

His letters home stressed the spartan aspect of his existence. 'At night I am in my lodging. I have hardly any other society but a folio book, a skeleton, my cat and my meagre landlady.'[9] He wrote to Bob Bryanton, a Trinity College crony, in a lighter mood: 'No turnspit gets up into his wheel with more reluctance than I sit down to write, yet no dog ever loved the roast meat he turns better than I do him I now address . . .'. After this pleasing start he gives a description of life in Edinburgh that suggests he is enjoying the social whirl. But even to Bryanton he admits that 'An ugly man and a poor man is society only for himself and such society the world lets me enjoy in great abundance.'[10]

That he left Edinburgh without a degree need not surprise us. 'In the first part of the eighteenth century [according to Kirkpatrick] men went to Edinburgh to study not to graduate.'[11] If he was going on to continental schools, why waste money printing a thesis in Edinburgh? A letter to his uncle, the Rev. Thomas Contarine, expressed his intention to return eventually to Ireland to practise as a physician: 'How I enjoy the pleasing hope of returning with skill and to find my friends stand in no need of my assistance.'[12]

He proceeded to Leyden and seems to have spent some time in Louvain, Paris and Padua during his travels. The golden age of medicine in Leyden had ended when Boerhaave died in 1738 and Goldsmith found the teaching there inferior to that of

Edinburgh but was impressed by Gaubius, the professor of chemistry whom Boswell later consulted. In conversation with Gaubius, Goldsmith spoke of Edinburgh and his teacher complained that whereas English students formerly favoured Leyden, they were now flocking to Edinburgh. He assumed that the professors there were wealthy and was surprised to be told that this was not so. '"Poor men," says he, "I heartily wish they were better provided for, until they become rich, we can have no expectation of English students at Leyden."'[13]

He intended to join the classes of Ferrein, Jean Louis Petit and Du Hammel de Monceau in Paris, where he attended Rouelle's chemistry lectures. Evidently these lectures were social as well as academic occasions, for he wrote, 'I have seen as bright a circle of beauty at the chemical lectures of Rouelle as gracing the court at Versailles.'[14] Nothing is known of his visits to Louvain or Padua, the latter famous now for its many distinguished alumni and professors, including Linacre and Caius, William Harvey, discoverer of the circulation of the blood (1628), and Andreas Vesalius, author of *De Fabrica Humani Corporis* (1543).

Goldsmith returned to England on 1 February 1756, a penniless, tattered vagabond. By the following year he had managed to set up as a physician in Bankside, Southwark, having meanwhile worked as an apothecary's assistant, a menial occupation for a university graduate in physic, if such he purported to be, and as a teacher or usher, a position which need not surprise us for in the eighteenth century an educated man could aspire to a plurality of posts. Whitley Stokes, for instance, was 'Medicus' in TCD and also Donegall Professor of Mathematics and Lecturer on Natural History.

Early days in medical practice are never easy and when a printer's workman, who was Goldsmith's patient, recommended him to Samuel Richardson, he found an entrée to the world of letters and to his real *métier*. Then, through Doctor John Milner, a Peckham schoolmaster, he was introduced to Ralph Griffiths, a bookseller and proprietor of the *Monthly Review*, and went up a step or two in Grub Street. Writing to his brother-in-law, Daniel Hodson, in 1757, the year he went to lodge with Griffiths, he stated: 'By a very little practice as a physician and a very little reputation as an author I make a shift to live.'[15] He could, of

course, have practised conveniently at the coffee-houses he fre-
quented and many of his letters bore the address Temple Exchange
Coffee-house.

An amusing letter to Bob Bryanton may suggest that behind
the mask of comedy academic recognition was actually coveted:

Do you know who you have offended? A man whose character may one of
these days be mentioned with profound respect in a German comment or
Dutch dictionary; whose name you will probably hear ushered in by a Doc-
tissimus Doctissimorum, or heel-pieced with a long Latin termination. Think
how Goldsmithius, or Gubblegurchius or some such sound, as rough as a nut-
meg grater, will become me. Think of that![16]

From these happy fancies he returned to the reality that faced
him – 'Oh Gods! Gods! here in a garret waiting for bread and
expecting to be dunned for a milk score!'

His financial plight impelled him in 1758 to accept a post as
physician and surgeon to a factory on the coast of Coromandel
with an annual salary of £100 and expectations of earning £1000
per annum from private practice. This engagement fell through
when the area he was destined for was taken by the French and
meanwhile, in December 1758, he was rejected at Surgeons'
Hall for the post of surgeon's-mate.

His wish to qualify as a surgeon's-mate does not necessarily
indicate that he did not then possess a medical degree. He may
have hoped to take a paid passage on an East Indiaman. He could
have failed for lack of indentures or because with the convinced
superiority characteristic of eighteenth-century physicians he
neglected to acquaint himself with basic surgical realities.

An Enquiry into the State of Polite Learning in Europe was published
in 1759. On 31 March 1763 he is referred to as MB in an agreement in his own handwriting with Dodsley and on the title-page
of *The Traveller* (1764) he is styled Oliver Goldsmith MB. At the
suggestion of friends, including Sir Joshua Reynolds, he again
embarked on medical practice in 1765, when the success of *The
Traveller* had brought him a certain renown which might possibly
attract patients.

He engaged a manservant and decked himself out suitably, or
so he thought, but Prior remarks: 'Transformations of this kind
in men who are more familiar with books than with common

life are often in extremes . . . '. This biographer gives us a picture of Goldsmith:

an exceedingly smart physician dressed [in a] conspicuous and expensive, though as appears from the fashion of the day, not an unusual medical garb. A professional wig and a cane, purple silk small clothes, a scarlet roquelaure buttoned to the chin.[17]

The second venture into practice was again unprofitable. For one thing he was temperamentally unsuited to it, unable to adopt a becoming gravity, complaining 'that he was now shut out from many places where he had formerly played the fool very agreeably', for another, he was probably quite incompetent, as is suggested by his management of the unfortunate Mrs Sidebotham.

This lady, a friend of his, sought his advice but his prescription so alarmed an apothecary that he refused to dispense it. Goldsmith would not alter it and an acrimonious argument ensued in which neither physician nor apothecary would give way. Nothing was left but an appeal to the patient but she, alas, forgetting friendship and valuing her health, took the apothecary's advice.

Greatly riled by the incident, Goldsmith quitted the house and later declared that he would cease prescribing for his friends, leaving himself open to Topham Beauclerk's sardonic humour. 'Do so, my dear Doctor,' Beauclerk said, 'whenever you undertake to kill let it be only your enemies.'[18]

In February 1769, accompanied by Dr Johnson and the Rev. Thomas Percy, later Bishop of Dromore, he visited Oxford University and was granted an *ad eundem* MB.

Doctors who desert medicine for literature do not, as a rule, parade their technical knowledge other than in the 'cut 'em ups' or medical novels. Goldsmith is no exception but he did poke fun at the profession. The 'Elegy on the Glory of her Sex, Mrs Mary Blaize' is a good example: 'Her doctors found, when she was dead/Her last disorder mortal . . . '.[19] The failure of the *Gentleman's Journal*, a fortnightly on which he worked (in company with Drs Kenrick, Bickerstaff and Hiffernan) led an acquaintance to remark that it had had an extraordinary death: 'Not at all, sir,' Goldsmith replied, 'a very common case; it died of too many doctors.'

His other medical colleagues in Grub Street were an Irish acquaintance, Samuel Glover; Tobias Smollett, the novelist; and James Grainger, MD Edinburgh, who had served as an army surgeon before establishing himself on Griffiths's *Monthly Review*. Smollett attacked Grainger's version of Tibullus but commissioned Goldsmith to write for the *Critical Review* in 1759. Grainger, whom Goldsmith met from time to time in the Temple Exchange Coffee House, introduced him to the Rev. Thomas Percy, later Bishop of Dromore.

He had acquaintances, too, among leading members of the conventional medical profession and acknowledged a tardy invitation to dinner at Dr (later Sir George) Baker's:

> Your mandate I got,
> You may all go to pot;
> Had your senses been right,
> You'd have sent before night;
> As I hope to be saved,
> I put off being shaved;
> For I could not make bold,
> While the matter was cold,
> To meddle in suds,
> Or to put on my duds . . . [20]

Dr William Hunter, a distinguished anatomist and man-midwife, was approached by Goldsmith on his nephew's behalf when William Hodson came to London, uncertain whether to go on the stage or to study medicine: 'The young gentleman who carries this is my nephew. He has been liberally bred and has read something of physic and surgery, but desires to take the shortest and best method of being made more perfect in these studies . . .'.[21]

William Blizzard (b. 1743) drained Goldsmith's manservant's empyema following a chest infection. He was one of the founders of the London Hospital Medical School, the professor of anatomy to the Surgeons' Company and was knighted in 1803. Sir William Blizzard still operated as an octogenarian and was one of the last professional men to attend patients in London's coffee-houses.[22]

'The Clown's Reply', written in Edinburgh in 1753, bears the stamp of neither literary nor medical promise, and throughout his dual career whatever clinical images appear are probably fortuitous. 'Now breaking a jest, and now breaking a limb!' And yet he does express instinctive psychological perceptions – 'the loud laugh that spoke the vacant mind' – and registers acceptance of the separateness and desolation of the creative artist:

> My shame in crowds, my solitary pride;
> Thou source of all my bliss, and all my woe,
> Thou found'st me poor at first and keep'st me so . . . .[23]

The solemnity of death is a hackneyed subject for poets, its easeful and merciful finality a proven reality for doctors, so one or both may speak in 'Threnodia Augustalis': 'Death, when unmask'd, shows me a friendly face, / And is a terror only at a distance . . . '.[24]

Writing to his brother-in-law, Daniel Hodson, Goldsmith referred to a '*maladie du païs*', the homesickness that in some degree he continued to suffer throughout his life and which emerged in *The Deserted Village*:

> In all my wand'rings round this world of care,
> In all my griefs – and God has given my share –
> I still had hopes, my latest hours to crown,
> Amidst those humble bowers to lay me down . . .
> I still had hopes, my long vexations past,
> Here to return – and die at home at last. [25]

He made inspired use of the pica of pregnancy when he wrote: 'My desires are as capricious as the big-bellied woman's who longed for a piece of her husband's nose.'[26] And no more kindly interpretation of senile dementia has ever been penned than that in his letter to Mrs Jane Lawder, referring to Contarine, his uncle:

He is no more the soul of fire as when once I knew him. Newton and Swift grew dim with age as well as he . . . Yet who but the fool would lament his condition, he now forgets the calamities of life, perhaps indulgent heaven has given him a foretaste of that tranquillity here which he so well deserves hereafter.[27]

Now and then he offered more technical data, as when adding a footnote to an article on Burke's *Essay on the Sublime and Beautiful*:

The muscles of the uvea act in the contraction, but are relaxed in the dilatation of the ciliary circle. Therefore, when the pupil dilates, they are in a state of relaxation, and the relaxed state of a muscle is its state of rest. In an amaurosis, where these muscles are never employed, the pupil is always dilated. Hence darkness is a state of rest to the visual organ, and consequently the obscurity which the author justly remarks to be often the cause of the sublime is often caused by a relaxation of the muscles, as well as by a tension.[28]

His reviews sometimes dealt with medical subjects. He dismissed *A Treatise upon Dropsies* as 'a quack-bill, lengthened out into the shape of a pamphlet'[29], regarded *A new Method of treating the common Continual Fever, and some other Distempers*[30] as 'absurd, both in theory and practice', and on the assumption that the 'Lisbon Diet-Drink' was a secret remedy asked: 'To what purpose then a long pamphlet on its efficacy?'[31] Dr D.P. Layard's *Essay on the Nature, Causes, and Cure of the contagious Distemper among the Horned Cattle in these Kingdoms* he reviewed at some length, giving descriptive details of the illness, its possible cause – 'pestilential effluvia, of a very subtle and active nature, taken in either by inspiration, or deglutition, first vitiating the fluids, then relaxing, and lastly, destroying the solids of the cattle' – and its treatment. Layard's therapy is credited with the cure of five out of seven cows treated.[32]

Léopold Auenbrugger's *Inventum Novum*, published in Vienna in 1761, introduced percussion of the chest, a valuable diagnostic method still in use. The medical profession was slow to recognize its utility but a perceptive anonymous review appeared in Newbery's *Public Ledger* on 27 August 1761 and has been attributed to Goldsmith by Ronald S. Crane.[33]

There has been just published at Vienna [the reviewer wrote], a Latin treatise with the following title, 'Leopoldi Avenbrugger, Medicinae Doctoris, in Caesarea regio nosocomio, nationum Hispanica Medici Ordinarii, inventum novum expercussione thoracis humani ut signo abstrusos interni pectoris morbos detegendi; Or, a new invention for the discovery of latent disorders in the breast, by striking the thorax; by Leopold Avenbrugger, M.D. &c.'

I have not, says our medical adventurer, been incited to this publication by an itch for writing, nor the delusive pleasure of speculation, but an experience of seven years has confirmed my opinion, and improved my practice in this discovery. He continues to observe, that the thorax (*or that part of the body which lies under the upper ribs and breast bone*) when struck by the tops of the fingers armed with a glove, sounds somewhat like a drum when covered with a woollen cloth; this sound is in every part pretty nearly equal except just over the heart. In lean men the sound is more perceptible than in fat, and the latter require a stronger blow to excite it. This sound he affirms to be one principal criterion of the state of the thorax, and in those who have a latent disorder there the difference of the sound is easily perceptible.[34]

The reviewer goes on to describe in some detail how to percuss the chest, adding a cautionary note: 'the lungs are often even in the most healthy state, found to adhere to the pleura, and in such a case, I fancy the sound would, in that part, deceive the practitioner' – an observation which led Saul Jarcho, an American medical historian, to suggest that Goldsmith's knowledge of clinical medicine was greater than is generally credited to him:

Goldsmith's review of Auenbrugger must be commended for several reasons. It is clear, instructive, and rather accurate. It is obviously based on a first-hand knowledge of the original text. It is conspicuously free from the bitterness and hostility which defaced a high proportion of the few notices that Auenbrugger received. Goldsmith's natural geniality and his remoteness from the medical politics of Vienna made it unnecessary for him to fear the new discovery. Unlike Auenbrugger's French translator, Rozière de la Chassagne, Goldsmith did not misconstrue percussion as a variant of Hippocratic succussion.[35]

This review, unfortunately, did not succeed in persuading British doctors to adopt Auenbrugger's diagnostic method, which was not widely used until revived in France by Jean-Nicholas Corvisart, Napoleon's favourite physician, in 1808.

The cordiality shown to Auenbrugger was not extended to Linnaeus, who is mentioned disparagingly in Goldmith's review of *A New and Accurate System of Natural History* by R. Brookes:

Should a Learner, for instance, desire to know something of the bird of Paradise, let him apply to the system of the great Swedish Naturalist, and there he will be taught, that it is a bird of the raven kind, for it has like it a cultrate beak, and setaceous feathers at the base: this, it is true, will give him but a very imperfect idea of the bird of Paradise, but a sublime idea of the Philosopher's learning. The truth is, the Swedes and the Germans, who of late have undertaken to improve Natural History, seem to err as the Schoolmen did of old; both rank the objects of the natural and ideal world under certain classes or categories, and when asked concerning any particular object, only tell you, to what class it belongs: and away they walk, filled with the vast idea of their own learned importance.[36]

To Mrs Bunbury (sister of the Jessamy Bride), who addressed him as 'my good Doctor', Goldsmith wrote: 'Pray, Madam, where did you ever find the epithet "good" applied to the title of Doctor? Had you called me learned Doctor, or grave Doctor, or noble Doctor, it might be allowable because they belong to the profession.'[37] A doctor is not mentioned in *The Deserted Village*; *The Vicar of Wakefield* contains a brief reference: 'Physicians tell us of a disorder in which the whole body is so exquisitely sensible that the slightest touch gives pain.'

Sir William Hale-White of Guy's Hospital, in a bicentenary tribute, insisted that Goldsmith 'was a physician of whom our profession may be well proud, for he wrote the best comedy in our tongue and Goethe said "It is not to be described the effect that Goldsmith's *Vicar* had upon me, just at that critical moment of mental development . . .".' Sir William had found no reference to medicine in *The Man in Black*; he mentioned Goldsmith's advice on the correct diet for children in *The Bee* but overlooked a passage on the endemic goitre of the Alps, 'where the inhabitants had each a large excrescence depending from the chin, like the pouch of a monkey'. Some acquaintance with physiology is evident in the *Critical Review* where voluntary movements are related to the cerebrum.[38]

The epilogue to *The Good-Natured Man* ('No, no, I've other contests to maintain; To-night I head our troops at Warwick Lane,') refers to a conflict between the licentiates of the College of Physicians and its governing body. The plays do not have a doctor in their casts but Sourby, 'the Grumbler' in the farce of that name, says: "'Yes, tell him that when he will, without costing him a farthing, I'll bleed and purge him his bellyful!'"[39]

The posthumously published *An History of the Earth and Animated Nature*, a work in eight volumes written between 1771 and 1773, was Goldsmith's most remarkable undertaking.[40] Richard Cumberland (a dramatist friend represented as 'a sweet-bread' in *Retaliation*), forgetting, perhaps, that as a medical student Goldsmith had sat under the experts in natural history of several nations, thought him unsuited to the task – 'he hardly knows an ass from a mule, nor a turkey from a goose . . .'.[41] Dr Johnson, on the other hand, predicted correctly that he would 'make it as entertaining as a Persian Tale'.[42] Goldsmith himself evidently welcomed the opportunity to earn £800 by engaging his talents as a compiler while indulging his taste for studies close to those he once described as 'the most pleasing in nature so that my labours are but a relaxation . . .'.[43] He signed an agreement with William Griffin, the bookseller, on 13 June 1769.

In the previous August he had met Horace Benédict de Saussure, a Swiss scientist, from whom useful information could have been obtained.[44] He may have profited, too, from conversation with Topham Beauclerk, who, according to Goldsmith, was 'going directly forward to becoming a second Boyle. Deep in Chymistry and Physics.'[45] Be that as it may, the more tangible source of knowledge was a heap of books requiring two post-chaises to move them when he went out to Selby's farm. He extracted information from many authors, including Jan Swammerdam, who, despite repeated discouragements, 'went on peeping into unwholesome ditches, wading through fens, dissecting spiders and enumerating the blood-vessels of a snail'. His major authority was the Comte de Buffon.[46]

Animated Nature was written for the general reader. 'Professed naturalists will, no doubt, find it superficial . . . '.[47] He proposed to avoid 'long Greek names . . . Indeed, few readers would think themselves improved, should I proceed with enumerating the various classes of the Coniethyodontes, Polyleptoginglimi, or the Orthoceratites.'[48] He admitted to having 'a taste rather classical than scientific' and his lovely images effectively edged out the plain prose of the would-be naturalist: 'Everything we see, gives off its parts to the air, and has a little floating atmosphere of its own around it. The rose is encompassed with a sphere of its own odorous particles . . .'.[49]

The world's great rivers attracted surprisingly appropriate metaphors –

The rivers of the torrid zone, like the monarchs of the Country, rule with despotic tyranny, profuse in their bounties, and ungovernable in their rage. The rivers of Europe, like their kings, are the friends, and not the oppressors of the people . . . [50]

Having devoted his first volume to the earth, its fabric, internal structures, caves and subterranean passages, mountains, rivers and oceans, the air and violent phenomena such as earthquakes and volcanoes, Goldsmith turns in the second volume to theories of the generation of man advanced by Hippocrates, Aristotle and others. The former regarded fecundity as proceeding 'from the mixture of the seminal liquor of both sexes' but Aristotle 'would have the seminal liquor in the male alone to contribute to this purpose, while the female supplied the proper nourishment for its support'.[51]

Steno and Harvey observed the importance of the ovaries; Fallopius described the *tubae uterinae*; Van Leeuwenhoek, using a microscope, found 'infinite numbers of little living creatures, like tadpoles' in the male ejaculate. The process of fertilization was not clarified during Goldsmith's lifetime and he did not exclude the possibility of spontaneous generation: 'later discoveries have taught us to be more cautious in making general conclusions, and have even induced many to doubt whether animal life may not be produced merely from putrefaction'.[52]

Following Buffon, he supplied a good account of the development of the embryo and cited the work of Malphigi, Haller and von Graaf. Parturition is described briefly – 'the infant, still continuing to push with its head forward . . . at last succeeds' – without recognizing uterine contraction as a vital function. 'The blood, which had hitherto passed through the heart, now takes a wider circuit; and the foramen ovale closes; the lungs, that had till this time been inactive, now first begin their functions; the air rushes in to distend them . . . '.[53]

The first months of infancy 'are spent in a kind of torpid amazement' in which the baby learns to correct the information supplied by its senses. 'In this manner a child of a year old has already made a thousand experiments; all which it has properly ranged, and distinctly remembers.'[54]

Animated Nature went into more than twenty editions, several abridgments, and was translated into Welsh. It really is as exotic as any Persian tale and, just as medicine finds its way into the court, the seraglio and the hovel, there are tokens of it in Goldsmith's volumes, the most unequivocal and direct his pertinent advice on deafness:

this disorder also, sometimes proceeds from a stoppage of the wax, which art may easily remedy. In order to know whether the defect be an internal or an external one, let the deaf person put a repeating watch into his mouth; and if he hears it strike, he may be assured that his disorder proceeds from an external cause, and is, in some measure curable . . . [55]

He dismisses as 'a vulgar error' the powers 'ascribed to the hinder hoof' of the moose as an anti-epileptic remedy, refuses to be over-credulous concerning the dangers of mad dogs but takes very seriously the problems faced by miners. 'Coalmines are generally less noxious than those of tin; tin than those of copper; but of all, none are so dreadfully destructive as those of quicksilver.'

A generality is articulated in the first volume which remains true today and still is largely unexplained:

Diseases, like empires, have their revolutions; and those which for a while were the scourge of mankind, sink unheard of, to give place to new ones, more dreadful, as being less understood.[56]

The air, 'a chaos, burnished with all kinds of salts and menstruums', conceals mysteries that Goldsmith, no less than his Irish contemporary Sylvester O'Halloran, found challenging. Goldsmith posed the vital question that remained unsolved pending the discovery of oxygen, so readily absorbed by haemoglobin.

All allow it to be a friend, to whose benefits we are constantly obliged: and yet, to this hour, philosophers are divided as to the nature of the obligation. The dispute is, whether the air is only useful by its weight to force our juices into circulation; or, whether by containing a peculiar spirit, it mixes with the blood in our vessels, and acts like a spur to their industry.[57]

Volume Five is devoted to birds, 'a beautiful and loquacious race of animals that embellish our forests, amuse our walks, and exclude solitude from our most shady retirements'.[58] The ostrich is useful medicinally:

The fat is said to be emollient and relaxing; that while it relaxes the tendons, it fortifies the nervous system; and being applied to the region of the loins, it abates the pains of the stone in the kidney. The shell of the egg powdered and given in proper quantities, is said to be useful in promoting urine and dissolving the stone in the bladder.[59]

The palatability of the pheasant is mentioned: 'when the old physicians spoke of the wholesomeness of any viands, they made their comparison with the flesh of the pheasant'.[60]

Culinary aspects of fish have been discussed enthusiastically – 'On the other hand, our physicians assure us that the flesh of fishes yields little nourishment, and soon corrupts; that it abounds in a gross kind of oil and water, and hath but few volatile particles, which renders it less fit, to be converted into the substance of our bodies.' This diversity of opinion led Goldsmith to favour eating 'our flesh in the ordinary manner, and pay no great attention to cooks or doctors'.[61]

An analogy is drawn between fish-eyes and the eyes of near-sighted people. Those whose chrystaline humour is too convex, or, in other words, too round, 'are always very near-sighted; and obliged to use concave glasses, to correct the imperfections of Nature'.[62]

The rattlesnake's bite is usually fatal but 'a decoction of the Virginian snake-root' may be tried; the viper's bite is relieved by the application of 'sallad-oil'.[63]

Serpents 'copulate in their retreats; and it is said by the ancients, that in this situation they appear like one serpent with two heads . . . '. For some days before coition, snails 'gather together, and lie quiet near each other, eating very little in the meantime. . . . They then softly approach still nearer, and apply their bodies one to the other, as closely as the palms and fingers of the hands, when grasped together. At that time the horns are seen variously moving in all directions; and this sometimes for three days together.'[64]

The louse is an odious enemy of men, 'for wherever wretchedness, disease, or hunger seize upon him, the louse seldom fails to add itself to the tribe, and to encrease in proportion to the number of his calamities'.[65]

'The Pthiriasis, or lousy disease, though very little known at present, was frequent enough among the ancients . . . The use of mercury, which was unknown among the ancients, may probably have banished it from among the moderns . . . '.[66]

By day the bug 'lurks like a robber, in the most secret parts of the bed . . . '. Doubtless, Goldsmith spoke from bitter experience when commenting on the frequent occurrence of bed-bugs in French and Italian inns. 'They grow larger also with them than with us, and bite with more cruel appetite.'[67] To destroy them the furniture must be taken apart and painted with corrosive sublimate.

Because of its therapeutic usefulness, the leech 'is one of those insects that man has taken care to provide . . . '. Goldsmith gives instructions for their application – 'take them from the water in which they are contained about an hour before, for they thus become more voracious' – and removal – 'care should be used to pull them very gently' – in the sickroom.[68]

★

According to Oliver Goldsmith's sister, Mrs Hodson, the poet was his mother's favourite child. Her comment has not yet, to

my knowledge, inspired a Freudian analysis of the poet's mis-
fortunes but something of a tradition of denigration exists. Stephen
Gwynn[69] called him 'the ugly duckling of English literature' and
Lord Macaulay sarcastically cast doubt on his medical degree in
the *Encyclopaedia Britannica* (1856): 'He had, indeed, if his own
unsupported evidence may be trusted, obtained from the University of Padua a doctor's degree.'

When Sir Ernest Clarke, former Secretary to the Royal Agricultural Society of England, addressed the Historical Section of
the Royal Society of Medicine in 1914 on Goldsmith's medical
education and qualifications he took exception to Macaulay's
scepticism: 'This attack I regard as wholly unfounded and mon-
strously unfair.'[70]

On the evidence of J.A. Andrich's *De Natione Anglica et Scota*
(Padua 1892), from which Goldsmith's name is missing, Clarke
accepted that the poet did not have a degree from Padua. He
thought it unlikely that a degree had been obtained from any
other foreign university but was impressed by a footnote in the
biography based on material supplied by Dr Percy, Bishop of
Dromore, prefixed to Goldsmith's *Miscellaneous Works* (1801): 'In
February 1769, Dr Goldsmith made an excursion to Oxford
with Dr Johnson, and was admitted in that celebrated university
ad eundem gradum, which he said was that of MB.'[71]

Sir Ernest then described how he had turned to 'a large bundle
of papers labelled "Goldsmith"', once in the possession of Bishop
Percy, which had been entrusted to his care. Among some sheets
in Dr Percy's handwriting he found the following, written in 1769:

Tuesday 14 Feby. I went with Mr Johnson and Dr Goldsmith to Oxford.
W. 15. We all dined in University College.
Th. 16. We dined with Tom Warton in Trin Coll.
Sat. 18. We all returned to Town.
N.B. On this occasion Dr Goldsmith was admitted as eundem gradum, wich
he said was MB.[72]

He had then sought the aid of Sir William Osler, regius professor of medicine at Oxford, who, when unable to find relevant
information in the official registers, set to work on the files
of local newspapers 'a sleuth-hound',[73] who extracted a news
item from *Jackson's Oxford Journal* for Saturday, 18 February 1769:

'Yesterday Oliver Goldsmith, Esqr, Batchelor of Physick in the University of Dublin . . . was admitted in Congregation to the same degree in this University.'

Sir Ernest accepted it as proof that Goldsmith possessed a Dublin degree granted between his return to England in 1756 and 1763, the date of his agreement with Dodsley. His arguments are persuasive but in the following year Dr (later Sir) Raymond Crawfurd, physician to King's College Hospital, London, addressing the same body turned Clarke's evidence upside-down and concluded that Goldsmith 'had no degree in medicine at all, other than that conferred by Oxford University in 1769, probably under a misapprehension'.[74] He asks: 'Did Goldsmith's buffoonery prompt him to use *Jackson's Oxford Journal* as the medium of an elaborate hoax?'[75]

On the occasion of Crawfurd's address, the president of the Section of the History of Medicine, Dr Norman Moore, physician to St Bartholomew's Hospital, stressed that Goldsmith, an Irishman, would have been imperfectly understood by the English. 'Goldsmith's honour and integrity were notified by the company he kept, that of Burke and Johnson.'[76] Later, Dr T.P.C. Kirkpatrick, TCD's medical historian, took Crawfurd to task, saying, 'Most people will, we believe, prefer to assume the integrity of Goldsmith's word rather than the judgement of Dr Raymond Crawford [*sic*]'.[77]

It must be conceded that Kirkpatrick had been unable to contribute positive evidence to assist Sir Ernest Clarke. 'Dr Kirkpatrick writes to me that he has already gone carefully through a file of Dublin newspapers from 1755 to 1768 without finding any trace of a medical degree for Goldsmith, though many of the degrees given by Trinity College are recorded therein.'[78] And in 1924, when prompted to return to the vexed question of Goldsmith's degree by Mr Justice Samuel's statement that the medical degree was obtained not at Leyden or Louvain but at Dublin, Kirkpatrick examined the records of the Royal College of Physicians of Ireland, where he was registrar: 'At that time the examinations for medical degrees in the University were conducted by the College of Physicians, and the names of those examined are recorded in the minutes of that College.' He found no evidence that Goldsmith had been examined by the College and believed then that 'the case for Goldsmith's medical degree in the University of Dublin must be regarded as not proven'.[79]

Scanning the biographies of Goldsmith, one gains a definite impression that the spirit of partisanship or the reverse frequently colours their authors' conclusions and that few of them have fully taken into account the imperfections of eighteenth-century records.[80] To look first at the latter, it is relevant to recall that doubt was cast on his possession of the BA degree – the official document could not be found and, 'misled by hasty examination of the records', Dr Wilson gave a wrong date. Prior eventually found his name, the last on a list of those granted access to the library, a privilege then reserved for graduates. He then learned that this supposed autograph had actually been written in by the librarian of the day.[81] Still on the subject of TCD's records, T.U. Sadleir has stated that 'A good deal of carelessness existed about 1740-80' in the keeping of the registers.[82] This persisted into the following century. When Burtchaell and Sadleir were preparing *Alumni Dublinenses*, their task was complicated by the discovery that James Henthorn Todd's *Catalogue of Graduates* (1866) contained many errors.

> Far be it from me [Sadleir wrote] to express in the slightest degree any criticism of the profound learning of the great Celtic scholar; I am glad to be able to say that the work was completed when he was suffering from failing sight with the result that the proof-sheets were never properly revised.[83]

The Abbé de Foere, chaplain to the English nuns at Bruges, explained in 1832 to Prior that at Louvain 'the annals of that period, including the period 1754–55–56, are wanting, and probably lost during the various disturbances our country underwent in the latter end of the last century'.[84]

The Rev. Bliss, registrar at Oxford, told Prior that there was no record of Goldsmith's *ad eundem* degree, adding that he had 'by no means ascertained that the Poet was not so admitted' for he had found 'a chasm in the Register of Convocation for 1769 from March 14 to March 18 . . . '.[85]

Goldsmith's attendance at the classes of Monro and others has not been questioned but actually no official record (other than the signature in the *Obligation Book*) now exists. My own enquiry in 1961 elicited the following reply from Charles P. Finlayson, Keeper of Manuscripts: 'I can find no record of Goldsmith's attendance at the University here. There are in fact no records of medical matriculation before 1762 so it looks as if some registers have gone missing since Prior's time.'[86]

Dr Norman Moore, commenting on Crawfurd's address, found it impossible to accuse Goldsmith of fraud in regard to the medical degree: 'Eighteenth-century university records were sometimes loosely kept. In Trinity College, Dublin, they were generally accurate, but it would be too much to assume that no omissions existed. Might not records have been omitted at Louvain and Padua, as at Oxford?'[87]

One must confront the negative and imperfect records with the positive evidence of contemporary opinion. Soon after his return to England, the acquaintances whom he looked up, such as Dr Sleigh, a fellow student at Edinburgh, urged him to practise as a physician, and, despite the failure of this venture, Sir Joshua Reynolds and others encouraged him, as we have seen, to try again in 1765, when literary success had brought him into prominence. By then he was widely known as 'Doctor' Goldsmith, a title which in the eighteenth century was not generally given to medical practitioners other than university graduates in physic.[88] His claim to the MB, as already mentioned, is seen in the Dodsley agreement and repeated in *The Traveller*'s title-page.

The ready acceptance of this claim by friends and enemies is important circumstantial evidence. Not even Kenrick challenged him.[89] Dr Johnson, who had failed to get the Dublin MA, by special favour never questioned Goldsmith's degree.[90] Sir Joshua Reynolds affirmed that Johnson held truth sacred 'whether in great or little'. Less scrupulous, Goldsmith told white lies. He threw them in the air, light as feathers, knowing that wherever they fell nobody was hurt.[91] 'I wish you would take the trouble of moulting your feathers,' Dr Johnson remarked.

Goldsmith told a lie, white or not, when he informed Bishop Percy that he had taken a medical degree at Trinity when he was twenty. But the author of the biography published by Swan in 1774 (possibly Dr Glover, who knew Goldsmith well) said that the poet 'took the degree of Bachelor of Physic at Louvain . . . '.[92] Having given the whole matter further thought, Kirkpatrick, lecturing in the School of Physic, did not doubt that Goldsmith described himself correctly as MB in the Dodsley document. Kirkpatrick believed that the degree may have been granted some time after 1759 and that it was given 'by the special grace of the Board without the performance of the usual acts. If it were given in this way, the grace might not be recorded in the books of the Senior Proctor.'[93] This was quite possible. It was, indeed, so common for Dublin University to grant medical degrees by 'special grace' in the mid-eighteenth century, that the College of Physicians lodged a protest. There are a number of famous men who had degrees that are not recorded. Richard Brocklesby, a schoolfellow of Edmund Burke, for instance, is recorded in Cambridge as 'incorporate M.D. from Dublin', but in TCD there is no record of either his degree or his attendance. Later he became FRCP and physician to Dr Johnson.

The provenance of Goldsmith's medical degree may be disputed but its validity is supported by the fact that Samuel Johnson accompanied him to Oxford in February 1769 when the *ad eundem* degree was granted. Dr Johnson would never have participated in the perpetration of academic fraud. Thus, the entry in *Jackson's Oxford Journal* is compelling evidence and Sir Arthur S. MacNalty, a prominent medical historian, recalled to me how delighted Sir William Osler was to find it.[94]

When I last visited the University of Padua, in 1989, I was pleased to see that a mural in the Hall of Fame accords Oliver Goldsmith pride of place beside William Harvey, attired in academic dress and with a symbolic parchment in hand.

Goldsmith's attacks on quacks and their advertisements and handbills in the *Monthly Review* may also be adduced in support of his rightful claim to a place in the faculty. If lacking a degree, he would hardly have had the effrontery to speak so scathingly of the 'pests . . . patronized by authority, consulted by all, promising all things, performing nothing'.[95] Nor, I feel sure, would Garrick have been so ill-mannered as to contribute a prologue with a medical metaphor to *She Stoops to Conquer* had there been the least doubt as to the playwright's possession of a medical degree:

> One hope remains – hearing the maid was ill
> A *doctor* comes this night to show his skill.
> To cheer her heart and give your muscles motion,

He in *five draughts* prepar'd, presents a potion,
A kind of magic charm – for be assur'd,
If you will swallow it, the maid is cur'd,
But desp'rate the Doctor, and her case is,
If you reject the dose, and make wry faces!
This truth he boasts, will boast it while he lives
No *pois'nous drugs* are mix'd in what he gives;
Should he succeed, you'll give him his degree;
If not, within he will receive no fee!
The college *you*, must his pretensions back,
Pronounce him regular, or dub him quack.[96]

Goldsmith was unable to attend a meeting of the Club on Friday, 25 March 1774. He took ipecacuanha wine as an emetic and at 11 p.m. sent for an apothecary who practised in the Strand. This was William Hawes, who, in the early 1770s, was attaining celebrity for his endeavours to resuscitate persons apparently dead from drowning, and had benefited from Goldsmith's encouragement and assistance.

Apart from a disfiguring attack of smallpox, the poet had escaped illness in his youth; the privations of the student period do not appear to have harmed him but, in 1762, he explained to his publisher that he had 'been out of order for some time past' and his work on Plutarch's *Lives* was held up. Ten years later he contracted a severe urinary tract infection and the *General Evening Post* reported the intervention of Mr Percival Pott. The surgeon's incision released a discharge of purulent matter, but the patient attributed his recovery to James's Fever-Powders, given under the direction of Dr James himself.

Arriving at Brick Court, Hawes found his patient with a violent headache and asking for James's Powder, which, to the apothecary's mind, 'was a medicine very improper at that time . . . '.[97] Hawes favoured rest, a mild opiate and 'two or three half pints of warm Mountain-whey' to effect sweating. He attempted to reason with Goldsmith: 'I told the Doctor, that his stomach was yet hardly settled from the operation of the emetic, and that his frame in general seemed a good deal agitated; and therefore the Fever-Powder would be more likely to act as a simple stimulant on the primae viae than as a febrifuge . . . '.[98] As Goldsmith remained obdurate, Hawes reflected 'that he was bred a Physician, and therefore it was natural to converse with him on the subject of his disorder in a medical manner; but his attention had been so wholly absorbed by polite literature, that it prevented him from making any great progress in medical studies'.[99] When his vehement entreaty failed to convince the poet, the apothecary warned him that if he took the fever-powder it was entirely without his approbation. He then obtained Goldsmith's reluctant permission to call in Dr Fordyce, a physician he had previously consulted.

George Fordyce, physician to St Thomas's Hospital, was born in Aberdeen in 1736. Despite an off-hand manner and carelessness in dress, he had a large practice. Holding the opinion that one meal a day was sufficient, he took no meal but dinner but, according to gossip, that meal was a liberal one. He sometimes drank too much and on one occasion at the bedside of a lady patient in his cups realized that he was unable to count her pulse. 'Drunk, by God!' he muttered. Next morning he received a letter from his patient (enclosing a generous fee) expressing her discomfiture that he had diagnosed her condition so accurately and entreating him to silence.[100]

Fordyce had lately been elected to the Club. On the evening in question he was to dine at the Turk's Head in Gerrard Street, where, as poor Goldsmith reminded Hawes, 'I should also have been, if I had not been indisposed.' But when Hawes's servant called to Fordyce's house in Essex Street, he found the doctor at home. He went to see Goldsmith at once and next day told Hawes that, despite their joint disapproval, Goldsmith had taken the powders.

When Hawes called to Brick Court on Saturday morning, Goldsmith was dozing; returning that evening, he learned from the manservant that despite repeated vomiting and loose motions, his master had persisted in taking James's powders.

I afterwards went into Dr Goldsmith's chamber, and found him extremely reduced, and his pulse was now become very quick and small. When I enquired of him how he did, he sighed deeply, and in a very low voice said, 'he wished he had taken my friendly advice last night' (meaning Friday night, the twenty-fifth of March): and this was all he said during this visit; for whatever other questions I thought proper to ask him, he appeared so much exhausted as not to be able to make any reply to them; and I clearly perceived he was so very weak and low, from the large and copious evacuation, that he seemed to have neither strength nor spirits to speak.[101]

Initially, Hawes had regarded Goldsmith's illness 'to be more a nervous affection than a febrile disease'. *Pulvis febrifugus Jacobi*, which he so strongly condemned, was a fashionable nostrum containing antimony.[102] Evidently Hawes had seen 'several Cases wherein this noted *Fever-Powder* had proved highly injurious'; its dangers were increased by the frequency with which it was given 'at the discretion of Old Women, or, at least, by those who cannot have the smallest pretentions to medical knowledge'.[103] If it were to be administered, Hawes reasonably insisted, it should be properly compounded by a competent apothecary; he deplored the fact that it was recommended daily in the *Public Ledger*.

A modern diagnostician would suspect that by 1774 Goldsmith had well-established and incurable kidney disease resulting from an ascending bladder infection and that his death resulted from uraemia and septicemia. Antimony could have been an aggravating factor, acting as a metallic poison if not excreted and, by increasing the vomiting and purgation, promoting dehydration, which in turn aggravated the renal failure in an already mortally ill patient.

When Fordyce saw that Goldsmith 'lay absolutely sunk with weakness', he decided to avail of the advice of Dr John Turton, whose opinion Goldsmith was known to value. The two physicians continued to meet twice daily at Brick Court[104] but in the early morning of 4 April the poet was seized by strong convulsions and soon expired. He was buried in the cemetery of the Temple. The exact site of his grave is unknown and the sole record in the register reads: '*Buried 9th April, Oliver Goldsmith, M.B., late of Brick Court, Middle Temple*'.

NOTES

1. Joseph Cradock (1742–1826) was the author of *Literary Memoirs* (1826). John Forster in *Oliver Goldsmith's Life and Times* (London 1877) describes 'little' Cradock as a young man of fortune who with his wife came to London from Leicestershire in the early 1770s, 'quite a private little Garrick' (vol. 2, p. 293). Goldsmith contributed a prologue for Cradock's tragedy *Zobeide*, which was staged at Covent Garden on 11 December 1771.
2. Arthur Friedman (ed.), *Collected Works of Oliver Goldsmith* (Oxford 1966), IV, p. 344.
3. He was Oliver Goldsmith's cousin; his letter to Dr Strean in 1807 is quoted by Father Kelly: 'My grandfather . . . has often told me . . . that

Mrs Goldsmith spent much of her time with her mother, Mrs Jones, then a widow, at Smith Hill; that Oliver was born here, in his grandmother's house, that he was nursed and reared here, and got the early part of his education at the school of Elphin.'

4. William Wilde in William White Cooper's 'Narrative of the Last Illness and Death of Oliver Goldsmith, M.D.', *Dublin Quarterly Journal of Medical Science* (1848), 31–6.

5. Michael Cox, 'The Country and Kindred of Oliver Goldsmith', *Journal of the National Literary Society* (1900), I, Part II: 81–111. John Knott, 'The Birthplace of Goldsmith', *Lancet* (1910), 1: 281; Rev. J.J. Kelly, *The Early Haunts of Oliver Goldsmith* (Dublin 1905), *passim*.

6. Goldsmith was 'remembered favourably by the celebrated Black'. Forster, *op. cit.*, vol. 1, p. 48.

7. Alexander Monro, for whom the 'foramen of Monro' is named, was succeeded by his son and grandson as professor of anatomy. The Monros held the chair for 126 years (1720–1846). Monro *primus* was Boerhaave's pupil at Leyden, as were Andrew Plummer and Charles Alston. The latter was appointed professor of medicine and botany by the Town Council in 1738. Plummer had a particular interest in chemistry. He recommended the waters at Moffat Spa and devised a pill of antimony and mercury known as 'Plummer's Pill'. John D. Comrie, *History of Scottish Medicine*, vol. I, 2nd ed. (London 1932).

8. Katherine C. Balderstone (ed.), *The Collected Letters of Oliver Goldsmith* (Cambridge 1928), p. 6.

9. *Ibid.*, p. 3.

10. *Ibid.*, p. 13.

11. T. Percy C. Kirkpatrick, 'Goldsmith in Trinity College, And His Connection with Medicine', *Journal of Medical Science* (1929), 142–62.

12. *Letters*, p. 7.

13. *Collected Works*, I, p. 309.

14. *Ibid.*, p. 300.

15. *Letters*, p. 27.

16. *Ibid.*, p. 38.

17. Sir James Prior, *The Life of Oliver Goldsmith*, vol. II (London 1837), p. 104.

18. Forster, *op. cit.*, vol. 1, p. 396.

19. *Collected Works*, IV, p. 367.

20. *Ibid.*, p. 384.

21. Autograph letter in Library of the Royal College of Surgeons of England.

22. R.M.S. McConaghey, 'Sir William Blizzard and his Poems', *Medical History* (1958), 2: 292. Blizzard's diction was pedantic. He rebuked a student who spoke of a patient having his distended abdomen 'tapped'. 'Pray, what publican was you brought up under? Always say "paracentesis abdominis" or "paracentesis scroti".' An indefatigable rhymer, his verses dealt with many subjects and it was his custom to write a

soliloquy annually on his birthday. In 1826, at eighty-three, noticing an irregularity of his pulse he composed the following lines:

> Poor heart! at length art grown weary?
> Else, why the wonted throb suspend?
> Or, why the pulse with feeble tone?
> Or, what alas! these signs portend?

23. *Collected Works*, IV, p. 303.
24. *Ibid.*, p. 344.
25. *Ibid.*, pp. 290–1.
26. *Letters*, p. 50.
27. *Ibid.*, p. 47.
28. *Collected Works*, I, p. 34.
29. *Ibid.*, p. 23.
30. *Ibid.*, p. 22.
31. *Ibid.*, p. 31.
32. *Ibid.*, p. 68–71.
33. Ronald S. Crane, *New Essays by Oliver Goldsmith* (Chicago 1927), pp. 64–8.
34. *Public Ledger*, 27 August 1761 (reproduced by Jarcho).
35. Saul Jarcho, 'A Review of Auenbrugger's *Inventum Novum* attributed to Oliver Goldsmith', *Bull. Hist. Med.* (1959), 33: 470–4.

An inn-keeper's son, Auenbrugger knew that a cellar-man could tell whether a wine-barrel was full or empty by tapping on it with his figures and realized that fluid could be detected in the chest by similar means. He supported his conclusions by experiments on cadavers.
    A genial personality, Auenbrugger wrote the libretto of an opera, *The Chimney Sweep*, for the Empress Maria Theresa.

36. *Collected Works*, I, p. 141.
37. *Letters*, p. 130.
38. Sir William Hale-White, 'The Bicentenary of the Birth of Oliver Goldsmith, MB Dublin & Oxford', *Lancet* (1929), 1: 1229–32.
39. J.W.M. Gibbs (ed.), *The Works of Oliver Goldsmith* (London 1885), II, p. 297.
40. Oliver Goldsmith, *An History of the Earth and Animated Nature*, vols I–VIII (London 1774).
41. A. Lytton Sells, *Oliver Goldsmith, His Life and Works* (London 1974), p. 131.
42. *Ibid.*, p. 174.
43. *Letters*, p. 7.
44. Sells, *op. cit.*, p. 122.
45. *Ibid.*, p. 146.
46. James Hall Pitman, *Goldsmith's Animated Nature* (New Haven 1924), *passim*. The medical texts consulted include works by Ambroise Paré, Frederik Ruysch and Hermann Boerhaave; Bryan Robinson's *A Course of Lectures in Natural Philosophy* (1739); R. Whytt's *Essay Upon Vital and Other Involuntary Motions* (1751).
47. *Animated Nature*, I, p. xiv.

48. *Ibid.*, p. 47.
49. *Ibid.*, p. 312.
50. *Ibid.*, p. 226.
51. *Animated Nature*, II, p. 16.
52. *Ibid.*, p. 22.
53. *Ibid.*, p. 47.
54. *Ibid.*, p. 62.
55. *Ibid*, p. 173.
56. *Animated Nature*, I, p. 330.
57. *Ibid.*, p. 332.
58. *Animated Nature*, V, p. 1.
59. *Ibid.*, p. 62.
60. *Ibid.*, p. 186.
61. *Animated Nature*, VI, pp. 182–3.
62. *Ibid.*, p. 163.
63. *Animated Nature*, VII, pp. 206–10.
64. *Ibid.*, p. 22.
65. *Ibid.*, p. 270. According to Pitman, Goldsmith's principal source of information about insects was Swammerdam, who 'like the bee whose heart he could not only distinguish, but dissect . . . seemed instinctively impelled by his ruling passion, although he found nothing but ingratitude from man, and though his industry was apparently becoming fatal to himself' (*op. cit.*, p. 18).
66. *Ibid.*, p. 274.
67. *Ibid.*, p. 282. Goldsmith's delightful description of the butterfly (*Animated Nature*, VIII, p. 30) is taken from Swammerdam: 'The butterfly, to enjoy life, needs no other food but the dews of Heaven; and the honeyed juices which are distilled from every flower. The pageantry of princes cannot equal the ornaments with which it is invested; nor the rich colouring that embellishes its wings.'
68. *Ibid.*, p. 311.
69. Stephen Gwynn, *Oliver Goldsmith* (London 1935), p. 13.
70. Sir Ernest Clarke, 'The Medical Education and Qualifications of Oliver Goldsmith', *Proc. Roy. Soc. Med.* (1914), 7, Part II: 88–98. Sir Ernest Clarke (1856–1923), a native of Bury St Edmunds, was a clerk in the Medical Department of the Local Government Board until 1881, when he moved to the Share and Loan Department of the London Stock Exchange. He was appointed secretary of the Royal Agricultural Society of England in 1887 and became Cambridge University's first lecturer in agricultural history in 1896. His avocations included music and bibliography.
71. *The Miscellaneous Works of Oliver Goldsmith, MB*, 2nd ed. (1806), vol. I, p. 36.
72. Clarke, *op. cit.*, p. 94.
73. Clarke, *op. cit.*, p. 95. The term was Osler's.
74. Raymond Crawfurd, 'Oliver Goldsmith and Medicine', *Proc. Roy. Soc.*

Med. (1915), 8, Part II: 7–26. Sir Raymond Crawfurd (1865–1938) was director of medical studies at King's College Hospital and registrar at the Royal College of Physicians. He contributed to Quain's *Dictionary of Medicine* and edited the fifth edition of Burney Yeo's *Manual of Medical Treatment*. He published *The Last Days of Charles II* (1909), *The King's Evil* (1911) and *Plague and Pestilence in Literature* (1914).

75. Crawfurd, *op. cit.*, p. 21.
76. *Ibid.*, p. 26.
77. Kirkpatrick, *op. cit.*, p. 159. T.P.C. Kirkpatrick was physician to Dr Steevens's Hospital and author of *A History of the Medical School in Trinity College, Dublin, The History of Dr Steevens' Hospital* and other books and articles.
78. Clarke, *op. cit.*, p. 97.
79. T.P.C. Kirkpatrick, *Lancet* (1924), 1: 51.
80. See also J. B. Lyons, 'The Mystery of Oliver Goldsmith's Medical Degree', *Irish Journal of Medical Science* (1962), 121–41; and *The Mystery of Oliver Goldsmith's Medical Degree* (Blackrock, Co. Dublin 1978).
81. Prior, *op. cit.*, I, pp. 98–9.
82. G.D. Burtchaell and T.U. Sadleir (eds), *Alumni Dublinenses* (London 1924), p. x.
83. *Ibid.*, p. xi.
84. Prior, *op. cit.*, I, p. 178.
85. Prior, *op. cit.*, II, p. 201.
86. Autograph letter C.P. Finlayson to JBL, 21 November 1960 and 14 January 1961.
87. Crawfurd, *op. cit.*, p. 26.
88. G. Graham, 'Doctor', *Lancet* (1957), 1: 264. According to this account the use of the term 'Doctor' to designate a medical practitioner did not become general until the nineteenth century and was then resented by university medical graduates.
89. Kenrick hated him and wrote after his death

> By his own art who justly died
> A blundering, artless suicide;
> Share, earth-worms share, since now he's dead
> His megrim, maggot-bitten head.

90. When the lack of an MA degree held up Samuel Johnson's appointment as a schoolmaster in 1738, Lord Gower asked a friend of Dean Swift to persuade Dublin University 'to send a diploma to me constituting this poor man Master of Arts in their University'. But Boswell wrote: 'It was, perhaps, no small disappointment to Johnson that this respectable appliation had not the desired effect . . .' R.W. Chapman (ed.), *Life of Johnson* (London 1970), pp. 96–7.
91. F.W. Hilles (ed.), *Portraits by Sir Joshua Reynolds* (London 1952), p. 77.
92. *The Life of Dr Oliver Goldsmith* (London 1774), p. 5.
93. Kirkpatrick, *op. cit.* (1929), pp. 142–62.
94. Letter from Sir A. S. MacNalty to JBL.

95. *Collected Works*, I, p. 24.
96. *Collected Works*, V, p. 103.
97. William Hawes, *An Account of the Late Dr Goldsmith's Illness* (London 1774), p. 1.
98. *Ibid.*, p. 3.
99. *Ibid.*, p. 20.
100. Sir Leslie Stephen and Sir Henry Lee (eds), *Dictionary of National Biography* (Oxford 1973), VII, pp. 432–3.
101. Hawes, *op. cit.*, pp. 6–7.
102. Brian Hill, 'Dr James's Powders', *Practitioner* (1953), 171: 71–5.

This nostrum is mentioned . . . by Dr Johnson; his sprightly friend, Mrs Thrale, took it on occasion; the poets, Christopher Smart, William Cowper and Thomas Gray are enthusiastic about its effects: 'I have great faith in its efficacy', wrote Thomas Gray; it is praised in Fielding's novel, 'Amelia', and in Southey's amusing 'Letters from England'. As for Horace Walpole, his correspondence leaves us in no doubt that James's powders were his favourite remedy. He has left it on record that he had such faith in them that he would take them even 'if the house were on fire'.

See also *Notes and Queries* (1925), 148: 351, 390, 412, 425; Dublin Hospital reports (1817), 1: 315–25. Extolling James's powders, John Cheyne, physician to the Meath Hospital, describes a clergyman who had several fits of apoplexy: 'But ever since he began to take James's Powder he has not had a single fit.'

The *British Medical Journal* carried advertisements for *Pulvis Jacobi Ver*, Newbery's in the 1860s and it was not deleted from the *British Pharmaceutical Codex* until the 1940s. It was still cited in Martindale's *Extra Pharmacopoeia* in 1952 as *Pulvis Antimonialis* syn. James's Powder.
103. Hawes, *op. cit.*, p. 9.
104. *Ibid.*, p. 8.

3

Milton's Dublin Editor: Edward Hill MD

EDWARD Hill is an established minor figure in the annals of Irish medical history, King's professor of medicine in Dublin University and several times president of the College of Physicians. Most accounts of Hill dwell on his aspiration to provide a new and adequate botanical garden and the feud with Dr Robert Perceval, who opposed him, and merely mention his unpublished edition of *Paradise Lost*. This perspective is correct from a vocational viewpoint but I shall present his professional career briefly, taking his literary interests as the focus of my attention.

I

The eldest of Thomas and Mrs Hill's seven children, Edward Hill was born on 14 May 1741 near Ballyporeen, a County Tipperary village now rejoicing as Ronald Reagan's ancestral place. The lad was tutored by a local clergyman until his father's death, when the family moved close to Cashel, where he attended a classical school daily until ready to go as boarder to the Diocesan School of Clonmel.

He entered Trinity College, Dublin, in 1760, was elected Scholar in 1763 and graduated BA in 1765. His intellectual brilliance was crowned by exceptional calligraphy; the task of writing out a testimonium for the Duke of Bedford was deputed to him by the Board, his reward five guineas. Instead of seeking a fellowship, a distinction thought to be well within his powers, he turned to medicine. He took the MB degree in 1771, proceeded MD in 1773 and was elected fellow of the College of Physicians two years later.[1]

Little is known of his medical practice but he is said to have been particularly interested in sick children.[2] Honours came to him swiftly. Before long Hill was lecturer in botany (1773), regius professor of physic (1781) – which chair he retained for 49 years, and physician to Mercer's Hospital. Directly and indirectly he was involved with botany, the importance of which in medical treatment at that time cannot be overrated. Just then, for instance, a Birmingham practitioner, Dr William Withering, having expertly selected foxglove as the active ingredient of a folk-cure, was about to introduce digitalis, a remedy still in daily use.

Hill was outraged to find that the physic garden available for him was a strip of rat-infested ground shadowed by the over-hanging branches of lofty elms and used as a dumping ground by the adjoining anatomy school, despite the supervision of an elderly gardener. He decided not to replace the old man when he died and approached the authorities for permission to use a vacant plot of ground at Townsend Street.

A *hortus sanitatis* was a traditional and, as Hill saw it, a necessary amenity for an eighteenth-century medical school; others, and particularly those who had experienced teaching methods in Edinburgh and elsewhere abroad, believed that the provision of facilities for clinical teaching was a priority. The School of Physic Act of 1785 elevated Hill's botany lectureship to a chair but funds were set aside for clinical lectures, leaving nothing for the garden.

Arrangements were made to reserve a ward for teaching in Mercer's Hospital. Later a house was rented in Clarendon Street but this proved too costly, and besides, Dr Perceval, who described Hill as 'a self-sufficient, vindictive gentleman, singularly obstinate in his own opinion', wished to establish an institution resembling the Edinburgh Royal Infirmary.[3]

The university and the College of Physicians eventually agreed to co-operate in order to provide a physic garden. The physicians offered an annual sum of £100 from Sir Patrick Dun's estate. The legality of the use of Dun's monies was disputed. Legal opinions were sought, subcommittees formed and the agreement made in 1793 was reversed in 1798 by the chairman's casting vote. Meanwhile, confident of success and with the provost's approval, Hill had leased a six-acre field at Harold's Cross, prepared to pay half the rent until such time as the ground was required. When the

College of Physicians withdrew its support, he decided to use his entire salary to fund the project but, in 1800, through the machinations of Perceval, the second School of Physic Act decreed that no person could hold two chairs and he was obliged to give up the chair of botany.

Finally, Hill went to law with the provost and fellows to recover his money. The case was tried at the King's Bench in March 1803 and Hill was awarded £618.[4] Subsequently he published *An Address to the Students of Physic* (1803), an apologia containing a promise couched in a Miltonic metaphor – 'Nor will I call from off the oblivious pool those Demons that have disturbed our primeval peace: those Spirits of malignant Passions, of Envy, Pride, Hypocrisy and mean Revenge.'[5]

II

An unrepentant humanist at a time when medical writers were using the vernacular increasingly, Edward Hill's ears were closed to pleas that in the medical faculty, examinations should be conducted in English. So long as it was in his power to influence matters, he intended to resist this change.[6] His preference for Latin as the conventional academic tongue reflects literary interests that led him to amass a splendid collection of books and to seek control of the university printing house.

T.P.C. Kirkpatrick's inference in his *History of the Medical School* that Hill needed increased space for his botany lectures is probably incorrect. However crowded the old Anatomy House may have been, it is unlikely that students would have been given the run of an area containing valuable machinery and types. And besides, Hill's comments indicate familiarity with printers' procedures. He complains, for instance, of an editor's 'Being unacquainted with the operations and rules of printing' and refers to Baskerville's 'hotpressed pages'.[7]

Hill was given the use of the Printing House by the Board for five years in 1774. The period was extended and during the years of his occupancy he was joined by Joseph Hill (the relationship, if any, is unknown), who in 1779 printed Anthony Vieyra's *Animadversiones Philogica*. This, as Vincent Kinane has pointed out, was the first of a series of scholarly works printed by Joseph

Hill. Books on mathematics and science dominate but the list includes the first book from the press to use Hebrew type (Buxtorf's *Grammar*, 1782) and the first work in Italian to be printed in Ireland (Boiardo's *Orlando Innamorato*, 1784), the production of which was supervised by Dr Hill, who bore the cost.[8]

But by printing political tracts of a seditious nature, Joseph Hill put the Board in an embarrassing position. A meeting was arranged between the Chief Secretary, Thomas Orde, and Provost Hely Hutchinson, who was asked to account for the printer's activities. Writing to the provost on 27 August 1784, Orde expressed concern regarding 'dangerous machinations in very dangerous quarters' and asked for Dr Hill's address.[9] On the same day, 'Dr Hill having . . . at ye Board resigned the use of the Printing House & delivered up the key, the head porter was order'd to take possession of the Printing House.'[10]

Nothing further is heard of the matter. Unlike a colleague, Whitley Stokes, who was deprived of a tutorship for favouring the United Irishmen, Edward Hill appears to have suffered no reprimand. One is inclined to see him as the printer's innocent associate but his *Address* inveighs against the Act of Union and an Assembly 'who were then preparing to close their political existence by the barter of the Rights, the Property, and the Peace of their Country'.

Hill's library, which he sold by auction in 1816, contained more than 1800 volumes. These included eighteen incunabula and 101 books printed in the first half of the sixteenth century. The wide range covered the Greek and Latin classics, Greek testaments, Hebrew Bibles, French and Italian literature.[11]

From his youth, John Milton's writings had, as Hill put it, 'obtained a preference' in his mind. 'When chearful and devoid of care, I have resorted to them for amusement and instruction, and they have contributed often to console me in the hour of sorrow.'[12] Having read many editions of the poetical works closely, he was increasingly concerned by the number of ill-conceived alterations he noticed, particularly in *Paradise Lost*. He finally decided to republish the second edition of *Paradise Lost*, printed in 1674 and embodying corrections made by Milton; to this end he collated it with several of the later editions. He was twenty-eight when he embarked on his avocational undertaking, which planned to include an index to the great poem. He finished it 44 years later in 1813. The dull task of transcribing in his fine meticulous hand a fair copy of the index was completed on Thursday, 29 July 1824.

The undated prospectus of *A New and Correct Edition of Milton's Paradise Lost* offered for 20s. a work in two octavo volumes 'handsomely printed on superfine paper' which was to be sent to press by Messrs Bentham and Hardy of Cecilia Street, booksellers, when a sufficient number of subscribers had been obtained. But for reasons to be explained later it was never published and the manuscript was donated to Trinity College by his granddaughter, Mrs Curtis of Portlaw, County Waterford, in 1874.[13] It has attracted little attention from literary scholars. Robert Bell, a former TCD alumnus and arts graduate, referred to it in 1839 as 'the most remarkable instance of devotion to the memory of a poet, to be found, perhaps, in the annals of literature', and called the Prolegomena 'a masterpiece of critical disquisition'.[14] It is a remarkable exercise in polemics, reminiscent in this respect of Dr James Henry's commentary on Virgil's *Aeneid*. James Henry read classics and medicine at Trinity College between 1817 and 1824 and may have been influenced by Hill.[15]

III

Hill's beautifully written manuscript comprises five copybooks containing a Prolegomena, a massive word-index to *Paradise Lost*, discussions on French translation and criticism, accounts of the engraved portraits of Milton and of plates used in the several editions. Tables of previous editors' errata are provided and an anthology of 'the Censures and erroneous judgements, which Writers have pronounced on Milton'. The fifth book contains Hill's notes on *Paradise Lost*. The alterations to be embodied in the new edition are written into his own interleaved copy of the 1674 edition.

He recalls in the Prolegomena how he became determined 'to restore to the World the *genuine Text* of our unrival'd Poet, cleansed and purified from every adventitious foulness . . . '.[16] With this intent he had read all the existing editions and could claim 'a knowledge of their peculiarities, more minute and critical, than any Editor has ever hitherto applied any pains to obtain'.

He indulges no hypothesis, removes nothing and spares no labour in the endeavour to provide a standard for future editions.

He did not hope to attain fame, his sole purpose 'to *preserve the Text intire*; and to absterge such blemishes as, from inadvertance or intention, may have been infixed upon it'.[17] Printers and editors are castigated for errors and omissions which blemish the editions of *Paradise Lost* published since Milton's death. The printers facilitated 'the mercenary usage of illiterate Booksellers'; the editors busied themselves in 'splenetic Criticism' and in 'the coacervation of futile, verbose Commentary'.[18] The third edition was hurried from the press in 1678 abounding in errors and Hill condemns the 'atrocious injuries its Editor has committed, even to the enormity of leaving out an entire line, the 659th of the XIth Book'.[19]

The folio editions (1688, 1692, 1695) incorporating the errors of the third edition down to the missing line made Hill very angry. The seventh edition (1705) also is judged to be inferior but, by some lucky casualty, the excluded line is reinstated. The eleventh edition is a worthless little book that should be thrown into a corner and Hill complains that 'the muddy Torrent of abuses and corruptions becomes still more turbid as it flows on, each successive Edition being polluted by an increase of new mistakes . . . .'.[20]

Editors selected for particular disapprobation include Elijah Fenton,[21] whose spelling and punctuation upset Hill, the Bishop of Bristol, Dr Thomas Newton,[22] dismissed for superficiality, and Richard Bentley, whose disrespect for Milton infuriated Hill, to whom *Paradise Lost* was 'an emanation from nothing less than an immortal mind'. Bentley believed that the proof-sheets of the first and second editions were never read to Milton, 'who, unless he was as deaf as blind, could not possibly let pass such gross and palpable Faults', and, though himself a septuagenarian, wrote pityingly that 'poor Milton in that Condition, with Three-score Years Weight upon his Shoulders, might be reckoned more than half Dead'.[23]

The Baskerville editions were praised for typographical beauty but Hill noted that John Baskerville, 'the boast of his country – and its shame', was obliged to sell his type, implements and the secrets of his art abroad.[24]

Then he expounded on the duties of the ideal editor:

A judicious and conscientious Editor will treat his Author, as the skilful Artist, who, to repair a Picture, the Work of some great Master, Rafaelo or Corregio, with light and expert touches of his pencil, fills up and hides its accidental flaws and fissures, but will not superinduce new tints or shades, to impair the perfections of the inimitable Tablet. Such an Editor will even spare some blemishes, which the Author, intent on more exalted contemplations, may have overpassed: and allows them to remain, as Spots may appear upon the disk of the Sun.[25]

When preparing his own edition, Hill took the second edition for model – a book 'worthy not of Cedar only, but to be inshrined in the rich-jewelled Coffer of Darius'[26] – consulting the first edition 'for the rectification of some few mistakes, which have been accidentally overlooked in the printing of the Second'.

Even the pointing did not escape Hill's attention: 'Nothing can more injuriously affect the sense of an Author's expressions than the wrong position of their points. Confusio punctis confunduntur omnia.'[27]

Towards the end of his abusive commentary he found praise for editions published in Dublin and based on the first and second editions – John Hawkey's edition (1747), 'issued in much purity from the Press of the University of Dublin', and another from T. Ewing – but may have thought this passage smacked of chauvinism and deleted it.

He wondered why the earliest editions were so little used:

The homely coarseness of their garb, devoid of every typographic decoration; (and which was soon outshone by the more imposing dream of specious Folios, or of other forms more trim from the printer's art, that usurped their juster rights,) may have principally caused this neglect; their mean appearance exciting but a feeble interest, and excellence being deemed commensurate with ornament.[28]

The index was completed after 'drudging labor' in 1813. Robert Bell described it as 'a marvellous exercise of human ingenuity – a task which ordinary powers could not have effected, and from which even great powers, associated with less energy, would have recoiled'.[29] Every word of the twelve books of *Paradise Lost* is incorporated and, where appropriate, subdivisions were used, e.g. read – participle; read – preterite; read – imperative; to read – infinitive.

Hill believed it would serve '*as an absolute preservative of its Text*, which, so long as this index, constructed on the genuine

Edition, shall continue in existence, can never more sustain abuse or corruption, without it being immediately and infallibly detected'. With its aid he was enabled to call 'the several tribes of Words' from 'their distinct recesses throughout the volume', examine the orthography and when necessary impose corrections.[30] Variations could generally be explained by Milton's use of different amanu-enses and Hill was not willing to accept the 'methodical design' suspected by other editors. This is 'chimerical' and he is prepared to impose uniformity.

Yet there are some cases that must be excepted, to which even this becoming Uniformity cannot extend. The participle *been*, for instance, when it is to be pronounced quicker, is always *bin*: And the pronoun possessive their, which is the Saxon hir with a t prefixed, is therefore universally written thir by Milton, except in a few instances, where, the Verse requiring a more lengthened and emphatical pronunciation, it is their, in the commonly-received form. These distinctions seem to have been too evidently marked by the Author to admit any alteration.[31]

Personal pronouns, he, me, she, we, ye, are written *hee, mee, shee, wee, yee*, when strong emphasis is required. Bell claims that Hill was the first to draw attention to Milton's use of orthographic variations to achieve variations of rhythm.[32]

Was he the first to embark on a Miltonic word-index? Possibly, but others shared the intention and the Rev. Henry Todd's edition of the *Poetical Works* (1809) contains an index which in addition to the general text covers Greek, Latin and Italian words.[33]

Hill approved of the German and Italian translations but said the French translations were 'nothing better than the attempts of presumptuous ignorance to do what far excelled the powers of that meager idiom to accomplish . . .'.[34] He shows, with an almost audible snort, that the Abbé Delille has introduced references to Isaac Newton, whose discoveries were not published until after Milton's death,[35] and charges him, in view of his substitution of thyme for fennel, with ignorance of what Pliny says '*of the gratefulness of the smell of Fenel to Serpents*' and finding a new employ-ment for Eve. 'With her *belles mains* the *jeune beauté* milks the goats and sheep! Why does he not make the Devil tell us how the *brillante conquête* managed her Dairy?'[36]

Hill's tirade against French translators is followed by a no less envenomed attack on French critics. They base their comments, he alleges, on inadequate translations, speak dogmatically on what they do not understand, and are inclined to attribute praise of Milton to 'national prejudice'.[37]

His survey of engraved portraits of Milton selects William Faithorne's (1670) as the best and condemns many others. He appends a selection of adverse criticism and mentions a copy of the 1674 edition of *Paradise Lost* in which the following lines were written in a contemporary hand:

> Milton his clubb hath cast at Paradise
> blind in his fancy as hee's in his eyes
> what need we all this bable of the spheres
> had right been don, he should have lost his ears
> this book shall nere procure him a good fame
> Eikonoclastes doth record his shame.[38]

Hill's copious notes occupy 240 pages of closely written script; I shall confine comment to a few in which we encounter the doctor in his legitimate role of natural scientist. Referring to the ancient river Adonis which yearly 'Ran purple to the sea, supposed with blood' (Bk I, 451), Hill suggests that 'the dust or farina of the flowers of the Juniper, Pine and Fir' may give the water its reddish tinge. He will not have it that Empedocles leaped into the flames of Mount Etna (III, 471); it is more likely that in his quest for knowledge the philosopher stood too close to the mouth of the erupting volcano and was suffocated.

The concept of the phoenix derives from the date tree, which stirs Hill's botanical imagination.

It is indeed not to be wondered at, that a tree so singular in its Nature should supply a subject for ingenious fiction. A tree which grows and flourishes only in the burning sands and burning winds of the torrid Zone; which retains its vigour and fruitfulness for Ages; And at length, when rather satiated with life than worn down by time, burns and dies, that a youthful Successor may spring up from its aromatic ashes, to bloom like the parent plant, and to run through an equally protracted period of Existence.[39]

'Greedily they plucked / The fruitage fair to sight, like that which grew / Neer that bituminous Lake where Sodom flam'd' (X, 560). The reference, Hill points out, is to the *Poma Sodomitica*, also called *Mala insana* or Mad Apples. They abound about Jericho, not far from the Dead Sea. They are attacked by an insect which turns the inside to dust leaving the skin entire.

The line 'Conspicious with three listed Colours gay' (XI, 866) leads Hill to mention that, Isaac Newton's analysis of light into seven colours being unknown to Milton, he accepts Aristotle's scheme.

Hill devotes a lengthy passage to Milton's lines on his blindness:

> So thick a Drop serene hath quench't their orbs,
> Or dim Suffusion veil'd (III, 25).

He explains that the *Gutta serena* or *Amaurosis*, 'called here a Drop serene, is a total extinction of Sight, without any perceptible injury of the form or constitution of the Eye, which still retains its brightness and transparency . . . '. The causes of the disease 'are of too subtile a nature for discovery'.[40] The older explanation of 'a cold, transparent watery humour that dropped upon the Optic Nerve and destroyed its function' is no longer tenable but it may be the result of 'a paralytic affection of the retina', a disease of the brain or pressure on the optic nerves.

The diagnosis of Milton's blindness remains uncertain; modern discussants add chronic glaucoma and detached retina to the disorders mentioned as possible causes by Dr Hill.[41]

IV

'Erinensis', a London journal's Dublin correspondent,[42] encountered Dr Hill at a social occasion in Mercer's Hospital, where, in the 1820s, Hill, then in his eighties, retained his position as physician and governor. Erinensis was a satirist who liked to lampoon Dublin doctors and their institutions but his portrait of Edward Hill may be genuine enough.

By accident he was dressed in the fashion; his coat, to the cut of which he has inviolably adhered for sixty years, presenting then as great a space between the hip buttons, as the most 'exquisite' of his neighbours. He talked of the Greek and Arabian lights of medicine, of Rhazes and Avicenna . . . and on entering the room, I thought that one of the figures of Hogarth's 'Examination at Surgeon's Hall' had descended from the wall, to converse with us on the topics of his day.[43]

Hill appeared to enjoy himself and Erinensis felt it must be a consolation to the physician's juniors, with the prospect of old age still remote, 'to behold successive cargoes of everything on the board descend into the hold of an octogenarian vessel that had sailed in safety across the quicksands of all the climacterics, and whose timbers still promised to withstand the assaults of many another gale'.

A survivor from the eighteenth century, Hill lived until 1830, by which time Robert Graves, William Stokes and Dominic Corrigan had taken leadership in Dublin medicine. His anachronistic presence would have lacked authority in face of innovations like the stethoscope. He must not be judged beside the young stalwarts of the 'golden age' of Irish medicine. He belongs to another era and illustrates a curious symbiosis involving medicine and literature; he stands alongside Paul Hiffernan, Oliver Goldsmith and Sylvester O'Halloran in a line continued by Robert Richard Madden, Sir William Wilde and George Sigerson in the nineteenth century.

Hill genuinely attempted to improve the Dublin medical school. He was outsmarted in the physic garden affair but his endeavours in this regard should be viewed in the wider context of Irish horticulture. In the last quarter of the eighteenth century, according to Charles Nelson, 'botany and horticulture were still slumbering here, and it was Edward Hill who stirred the "sleeping beauty"'.[44] His Miltonic manuscript is a polemical *tour de force*; whether it possesses intrinsic merit is a question to address to literary scholars, who seem to have passed it by. William R. Baker merely mentions Hill's interleaved and annotated copy of the second edition of *Paradise Lost* in his monumental biography of Milton.[45]

E.J. Arnold[46] has presented him as the hero of 'a drama of unrecognised talent'. Hill's correspondence,[47] recently acquired by Trinity College, indicates that until 1816 he planned to print the edition personally. When he wrote to Dr Phipps, registrar at TCD, on 22 January 1816, he referred to the work 'which it was my intention to execute under my own inspection in my own House, that the Edition, if God permits the accomplishment, may appear with faultless accuracy'. But circumstances had made him decide to leave his present abode, 'where every object brings painful associations to my remembrance; and which is much too spacious for my family, now reduced almost to an Individual'.[48]

He intended to move to York Street and sought the Board's permission 'to be allowed to perform my work in the University Printing House, which now, as I am informed, lies waste and unoccupied'.[49]

As the College minutes do not refer to Hill's request, it seems unlikely that he was allowed access to the Printing House. And yet, as we shall see, he did have a printed copy of Milton's text to send to Taylor in 1824.

Six years later we find Hill writing to a London publisher, Joseph Butterworth MP, and recounting how, since boyhood, his growing interest in *Paradise Lost* was accompanied by increasing indignation at 'the perverseness of misjudging Editors', until he became determined to republish 'the genuine edition of 1674, with that care and circumspection which I imagine that Milton would have exerted, had he lived to give another Edition of his divine Work'. He explained that initially his intention was directed exclusively to *Paradise Lost* but now he wished to publish 'the other poetic works also of Milton, after their *primitive Editions*, but without Annotations'. If his project appealed to Butterworth he would arrange to send him 'by some safe hand the MS of my Prolegomena; which contains, among other topics unnoticed by any former Editor, a History of the *Paradise Lost*, and of the vicissitudes of its fortune through its several Editions'.[50]

Butterworth expressed interest – 'If you could send it by Post it would come safer and more direct than by any private hand' – and reminded the doctor 'that we are chiefly in the Law Department, but such a work as yours renders us very desirous of affording any aid in our power, in honor of our immortal Bard, and for the benefit of the public'.[51]

Hill may have distrusted the postal service for he committed his Prolegomena 'to the care of a Gentleman', informing Butterworth accordingly on 4 July 1822. He envisaged an edition in three tomes; 'The Index will occupy one; And the Preface and Text of the *Paradise Lost*; My Notes, and the other additional matters; together with the *Paradise Regained*, and the remaining Poems of Milton, will be divided in the best manner between the other two.'[52]

Unfortunately, as Hill explained in February 1823 to William B. Taylor, a young Dublin friend who was studying law in

London, Butterworth had displayed the caution so necessary for publishers. 'Mr Butterworth does not find it consistent with his course of business to attempt the Edition of Milton, my design of which is more extensive than he imagined, and consequently more expensive. So that we must take other views . . . '.[53]

Butterworth's terms, had Hill bothered to consider them dispassionately, were by no means unreasonable for an academic venture. He offered to bring out the edition at his own expense in a less elaborate format and share the profits with the editor. But Hill expected to receive adequate payment for his copyright and he now authorized Taylor to communicate with 'such of those extensive printers as you may think proper . . . '. By April he was negotiating through Taylor with Thomas Cadell, a publisher in the Strand, and explaining to his agent, 'I fear nothing from Critics and Reviewers; every vain thought of popular applause is lost in my Ardent fondness for the Great Poet; and I despise the paltry artifice of *Book-making*.'[54]

Cadell intimated that Hill was not sufficiently explicit as to what he expected for his copyright. The publisher thought the committee which considered the matter would not pay a thousand guineas for the work, not 'from any deficiency in it but from the depressed state of the book trade at present'. If Hill would state the exact amount he wanted and arrange for the whole manuscript to be viewed, 'it would be the most certain way of arriving at a satisfactory conclusion'.[55]

Encouraged by Cadell's practical approach, Hill began to prepare a fair copy of the manuscripts. 'I do assure you [he told Taylor] that my present task in which no one can assist me is very arduous . . . But however I am not of a temper to be intimidated by difficulties; and with the permission of the Almighty, it shall be completed. I have no intention to chaffer about terms. The liberality with which the London Publishers promote works of erudition and taste, gives me a perfect confidence and security on that point.'[56]

When Cadell communicated with a Mr Rivington, 'one of the company of booksellers who publish Milton's work', the latter promised that when he knew exactly 'what number of Volumes the work would properly occupy, and also the remuneration required', he would call his group together and show them a specimen of the work and Hill's proposal. Then 'they would very soon decide whether or not they should undertake the work'.[57]

Hill worked assiduously at the transcription and towards the end of January 1824 he was ready to send Taylor what he had accomplished: 'That is, half of my Index; a Volume of Notes; and a printed Copy,[58] the text of which is most minutely conformed to that of the primitive, And authentic Edition, purged of their typographical anomalies, and of whatever palpable errors might be found throughout the entire of Milton's Poetical Works; in fine a Copy pure and faultless, and such as never yet has been presented for publication.' The remainder was to follow in due course – 'We shall soon see whether the Miltonic Committee will prefer the perpetuation of error and the blunderings of presumptuous Commentators, most injurious to Milton, to the adoption of an Archetype that retrieved his original purity and splendor.'[59]

By mid-November 1824, Taylor had received six volumes from Hill; these included the second volume of the index, the first half of which had not yet been despatched for its expected bearer had not proceeded on his journey, and returned it to Hill, who was still undecided as to the payment he should demand for his copyright – 'I am so entirely unacquainted with the book-selling trade, that I cannot rate the Value of my own literary work, except by comparison. – When such sums are paid for perishable Novels. – When a French imposter could receive *one thousand pounds* for a vile travesty of Milton . . . I shall think it very strange if my vindication of the abused Poet and effectual restoration to his native splendour, shall be despised.' He was prepared to leave the decision to the booksellers but expected to be treated with respect.[60]

A letter written by Hill to Taylor on 27 January 1825 has not survived but on 12 May he urged Taylor that should he 'encounter in any treaty a disposition to trick or chaffer' on the part of the booksellers he must refuse to deal with them. He sensed that the negotiations were not going favourably. 'Though these *liberal Miltonians* may join in "synod unbenign",[61] others, perhaps, may be found to rise in opposition to them, and adopt proposals, which will, to a certainty, prove highly profitable, as the publication must absolutely supersede all antecedent Editions.'[62]

As June passed, he continued fatalistically to await a decision: 'Though I believe it is not likely that anything satisfactory to me can arise in the business – Nor do I care.'[63]

Early in July, Taylor confirmed that the publisher had decided not to proceed with the edition: 'I cannot express the regret I feel on this result of so much mental and physical exertion . . .'.[64]

Hill did not respond to the news immediately but on 13 October 1925 he informed Taylor that the most satisfactory way of returning the manuscripts was to send them by parcels 'properly packed and directed *For Mr Mullen, Bookbinder, Nassau Street, Dublin'*.[65]

He confirmed the safe arrival of a consignment of manuscripts in November, 'but that mode being, as I think, too expensive, we may rest awhile till something better occurs'.[66]

After minor misadventures, the rest of the manuscript reached him. The last parcel was entrusted to Alderman C. Archer of Dame Street, Dublin, early in January 1826 by Taylor but Hill noted: 'I received not these MSS – 2 Vols of Index & Book of Notes, till March 10th – being retained by Mr Archer, without informing me of his having them.'[67]

He thanked Taylor on 15 May for his help: 'I have received *all my MSS*, which were troublesome to you so long; And am soliciting the University, who I am in expectation will aid me in the publication of them. 'Twas a lucky chance that we fail'd in our negociation with the Miltonians, an illiterate herd . . .'.[68]

Surprisingly, Taylor (an apt pupil perhaps) felt likewise and hinted at secret offers:

I quite agree with you in thinking it fortunate that the 'illiterate herd' who *obfuscate Milton*, did not get hold of your papers, the preference instinctively given by that class of persons, to dullness and dunces, has at last brought ruin, and bankruptcy upon themselves, as the natural consequence of their folly; Two or three of those semibarbarian publishers offered me their *bills* of Exchange at six, nine and twelve months, in payment for your work, but I happened to know that those persons were tottering and I declined accepting what they were pleased to call 'a generous offer!'[69]

Hill wrote to the provost on 5 December 1826: 'The in-decision on my supplicatory address for aid to accomplish an Edition of the *Poetical Works of Milton*, has painfully depressed my spirits . . .'.[70] Next he offered the Board on 27 June 1828 'for their acceptance, all the Books & M.S.S. relating to my design, without any reservation whatever, or prospect of future gain or pecuniary return'.[71] Finally, a Dublin firm, Messrs Bentham and Hardy of Cecilia Street, agreed to publish the edition by subscription.

The prospectus of *A New and Correct Edition of Milton's Paradise Lost* in two volumes on superfine paper, price twenty shillings, was printed as a tasteful leaflet and among those who acknowledged its receipt was the Lord Lieutenant, the Marquis of Anglesey, who promised to subscribe. Hill sent twenty copies of the prospectus to his son, the Rev. William Hill of Mothel Glebe, County Waterford, warning him not to distribute them uselessly. 'Give them to none but respectable people, of *fixt residence*; that when the work is finished may be easily found.'[72]

Before long he had a list of 125 subscribers, which included many state and Church dignitaries in Ireland, while from Oxford University the Rev. Drs Bandinel and Bliss, librarian and registrar respectively, pledged their support. Even so the publishers hesitated to send the manuscript to the press.[73]

According to his son, Edward Hill continued his work on Milton 'to within a year of his decease in October 1830, writing over again several times, with unparalleled patience, that immense mass of matter'.[74] That his pertinacity was not rewarded seems blatantly unjust but the seeds of this infelicity were self-nurtured.

Arnold suggested that the tirade against editors and booksellers in Hill's prospectus discouraged potential subscribers.[75] This is unlikely and besides we have seen that Joseph Butterworth was prepared to publish the edition; L. Prowitt of Bond Street made a similar offer but Hill insisted on payment for his copyright. The commercial publishers may have found him as unyielding as his opponents in various controversies had done. And the expectation of help from his Alma Mater did not materialize, possibly because his record made the Trinity dons wary of the vituperative scholar[76] whose character in his last decade bordered on the eccentric.

From February 1820 he had undertaken the duties of Dun's librarian in the College of Physicians, a post which necessitated resigning his fellowship of the College as the post carried a stipend of £70 ('provided he shall furnish the necessary fuel for such Library and lecture-room') and in his account of Hill at this period

Kirkpatrick wrote: 'We can picture the old man devoting the time he had to spend in the Library to the compilation of his index to the "Paradise Lost", and resenting the intrusion of readers who interrupted his work.'[77]

On St Luke's Day, 1826, T.H. Orpen was elected librarian and Kirkpatrick has described what followed:

Having ceased to be Librarian, Hill ceased also for the time to have any official connexion with the College. He evidently expected to be restored to his Fellowship, as was the custom; but, as nothing was done, he wrote on December 2nd, 1826, asking to be summoned to the meetings of the College as a Fellow, and threatened an appeal to the Visitors if his request was not granted. The Fellows do not appear to have been anxious for his presence in the College . . . Kindlier feelings, however, prevailed later on, and in January 1827 he was proposed as a Fellow. On April 23rd 1827, his name came before the College for ballot, and he received eight white and seven black beans. The result shows that he still had enemies in the College, but he was re-elected to his Fellowship.[78]

Hill came to the College regularly and played a useful part in the management of the trust estate. His last attendance was on 25 May 1829 but he was present at the governors' meeting in Mercer's Hospital on 28 August 1830.[79]

After his death on 31 October, the Milton papers passed into the possession of Parson Hill,[80] whose parish duties, or so he affirmed, made it impossible for him to go to London in search of a publisher. In 1836, however, he accepted an offer from Richard Brennan, a surgeon and apothecary in nearby Carrick-on-Suir, to act as his agent on a profit-sharing basis.[81] A year later, not having heard from Brennan, he called to his house. The surgeon was not at home so he wrote to him expressing anxiety – 'hints and surmises have been thrown out to me' – and demanding a written answer as to the whereabouts of the work. If the quest for a publisher was fruitless, he asked 'that you will now consider it high time to fulfill your reiterated promise of returning it to me'.[82]

Subsequently he learned that Brennan had not gone to London in person but sent the manuscripts to 'the celebrated Mr Thomas Moore, who admired them very much'; they were shown to a number of publishers and sent by a Mr McCabe, 'to whose care Surgeon Brennan had entrusted them', to Cork-born Robert Bell, to whom they must have been like unexpected treasure.[83]

Bell, an established literary figure in London, was writing a life of Milton for Lardner's *Cyclopaedia of Biography*. He added an outline of their contents to his own work but said: 'I do not feel justified in entering into any closer examination of Dr Hill's inquiries, because I hope they will yet be given to the world . . .'. He was enchanted, too, by Hill's beautiful script: 'They are written in an exquisitely small, diamond hand, with a uniformity, brilliancy and accuracy that might justify a comparison with some of the beautiful illuminated writings of the middle ages . . .'.[84]

William Hill established his ownership of the manuscripts by correspondence with Bell but agreed that for the present the latter should hold them and discuss them with any interested parties. He expressed a wish 'that all connexion between me and Surgeon Brennan in this matter shall now terminate'. Nevertheless, it was Brennan who returned the work to the Rev. Hill in 1845.[85] Meanwhile, Taylor had offered to buy the manuscripts in 1842 but Hill was uncertain of their value.

Edward Hill's grandson, who owned the manuscripts after the Rev. William Hill's death, was the last person to seek their publication.[86] With this in mind he wrote to Mr (later Sir) Anthony Panizzi, the Italian-born librarian at the British Museum: 'My great wish and ambition would be to see the work published . . .'.[87] He would give it to anybody who could achieve this and share the profits with him. Alternatively, he would be prepared to sell the manuscripts at a reasonable price. Obviously he rather hoped that Panizzi would value them. The latter's reply has not survived but he may have been too wise in the ways of the world to venture a judgment on the monetary worth of Edward Hill's life's work or to attach a price-tag to the priceless.

NOTES

1. T.P.C. Kirkpatrick, *History of the Medical School in Trinity College Dublin* (Dublin 1912), pp. 164–5.
2. James Wills (ed.), *Lives of Illustrious Irishmen*, vol. 6 (Dublin 1847), p. 472. His son, the Rev. William Hill MA, of Mothel Glebe, wrote: 'No physician of his time paid much attention to the Diseases of Children, his practice among them was most extensive, and it is much to be regretted, that he did not write on the subject for the benefit of posterity.'
3. J.D.H. Widdess, *A History of the Royal College of Physicians of Ireland* (Edinburgh 1963), pp. 89–91.

4. TCD Mun/P/1/1271. When the action taken by Hill against the provost and fellows went to arbitration it was decided

> that there is due and owing to the said Edward Hill the Plaintiff by the said Provost and Fellows the sum of Six hundred and eighteen pounds nineteen shillings and ninepence halfpenny which included the difference between the amount of the Plaintiff expenditure on the Botany Garden and the sums already paid to him by the Defendants together with the rent which will accrue for that moiety of the Lands called the Botany Garden on the first day of May next . . . And we do award . . . that plaintiff is to take the lease of the said Garden off the hands of the Defendants together with all Buildings and Materials thereon to his own use for ever hereafter.

5. Edward Hill, *An Address to the Students of Physic relative to the School of Physic in this Kingdom* (Dublin 1803), p. 13.
6. Kirkpatrick, *op. cit.*, p. 237.
7. *Ibid.*, p. 148.
8. Vincent Kinane, 'The Dublin University Press in the Eighteenth Century'. Thesis submitted for Fellowship of the Library Association of Ireland, 1981.
9. TCD MS. Donoughmore papers C/1/181.
10. TCD Mun/V/5/5.
11. *Dr Hill's Library: A Catalogue* (Dublin 1816). Hill's Library ('One of the most valuable, curious, and splendid collections of Books ever brought to Sale in Ireland', according to the auctioneer) contained 1811 items. The sale was held at the professor's residence, 8 Harcourt Street, on Monday, 1 July 1816 and subsequent days. 'This truly valuable collection has been the pursuit and principal care of the Doctor for many years past . . . the Classics are of the first and finest order. Nearly all the Elzevirs and Octavo Variorums, are mostly bound in Vellum.'
12. TCD MS. 629. 1.1.
13. TCD MS. 629. 1–5.
14. Robert Bell, 'John Milton' in *Eminent Literary and Scientific Men*, vol. I (London 1839), pp. 251–6.
15. See John Richmond, *James Henry of Dublin* (Blackrock 1976) and J.B. Lyons, *Scholar & Sceptic* (Dublin 1985).
16. TCD MS. 628. 1.28.
17. TCD MS. 629. 1.3.
18. TCD MS. 629. 1.4.
19. TCD MS. 629. 1.6.
20. TCD MS. 629. 1.10.
21. TCD MS. 629. 1.9. Hill believed that Fenton's edition (1725) stood

> conspicuous among the worst that have appeared . . . no Printer or Publisher has ever laboured with more sinistrous diligence, than he has shown, to distort and inquinate the Text of this great Work. In accession to his more material defects, having adopted, for his private habit in writing, some very absurd peculiarities in his Orthography and mode of pointing; Procrustes-like he mangles his ill-fated Author, to adapt his dislocated members to his own unhappy manner; thereby most in auspiciously consulting for his reputation of classic elegance and accuracy.

22. TCD MS. 629. 1.10. 'Let his Erudition stand acknowledged; but that he wanted sagacity, and was deficient in elegance of taste, and clearness of judgment, his performance in this Edition, at least, will give the strongest grounds to apprehend.'

23. TCD MS. 629. 1.9. Bentley, Master of Trinity College, Cambridge won many controversies and outwitted the fellows with whom he feuded for more than thirty years. He died at eighty when Hill was a year old. Had they been contemporaries he would probably have treated the physician as a light-weight but the *DNB* sides with Hill, observing that Bentley's edition of Milton's *Paradise Lost* (1732) 'has the faults of [his] classical criticism in a senile form' and none of his merits.

     A brilliant humanist, Bentley concluded from his study of Homeric metre that a letter (the 'digamma') was missing from the later Greek alphabet. Gerald Griffin (author of *The Wild Geese* and *The Dead March Past*) recalled how Tom Kettle, seeing Mahaffy crossing College Park, head bent in thought, said, 'There goes Mahaffy looking for the lost digamma.'

24. TCD MS. 629. 1.11.

25. TCD MS. 629. 1.14. Hill insisted that 'The business of an Editor' was not to amass line upon line of comments and illustrations aggravating 'the oppressive burden of that species of writing' under which the classics are overwhelmed.

26. TCD MS. 629. 1.13.

27. TCD MS. 629. 5.5. Hill takes the hapless Dr Pearce to task for removing the question mark that should follow *And what is else not to be overcome?* and substituting a semicolon. He teases out over four pages how the point of interrogation clarifies the meaning and how one is left floundering without it, appealing for support to the Latin versions of Hogg, Trapp and Dobson (the latter led into error by Pearce) and to F. Mariottini's 'excellent Italian translation'. He scolds Pearce, whose alteration 'actually deprives this passage of all its energy, and lowers it to a tame and common sentiment, which excites neither interest nor passion . . .'.

28. TCD MS. 629. 1.14.

29. Bell, *op. cit.*, p. 254.

30. TCD MS. 629. 1.25. 'This Index resembles that which *Erythraeus* digested for the Aeneid, but it is infinitely more minute, comprehending every monosyllable, and even every monosyllabic letter in the P l.'

31. TCD MS. 629. 1.25.

32. Bell, *op. cit.*, p. 254.

33. Rev. Henry J. Todd (ed.), *The Poetical Works of John Milton*, vols I-VII with verbal index to the whole of Milton's poetry (London 1809). See also Guy Lushington Prendergast, *A Complete Concordance to the Poetical Works of Milton* (Madras 1857); Charles Dexter Cleveland, *Concordance to the Poetical Works of John Milton* (London 1867); William Ingram and Kathleen Swain (eds), *A Concordance to Milton's English Poetry* (Oxford 1972) – the last-mentioned concordance was generated by an IBM computer at the University of Michigan.

Cleveland's preface refers to Todd's 'Verbal Index', in which he found 3362 mistakes. Of his own index, which took over three years to compile, he wrote:

> When I say it is an 'Index *to all the poems*,' I do not mean to say that it is an Index *to all the words* in those poems. There are many words which it would be absurd to notice in an Index: for instance, the *articles;* most of the pronouns . . . all the conjunctions; many *adverbs*; most of the *prepositions* and such *adjectives* and *adjective-pronouns* as present no striking idea . . .

Hill's index does include them, the conjunction 'and' claiming eight columns of closely written page numbers.

34. TCD MS. 629. 4.1. Hill believed the Latin version by Hogg, Trapp and Dobson was 'written for the learned' and must remain secluded; the Portuguese version had not been seen by him nor could he say if a Spanish version existed; neither had he seen Theodore Haake's Dutch version but had been told that John Thorlakson had translated it into Icelandic.

35. TCD MS. 629. 4.13.

36. TCD MS. 629. 4.12. 'For this travesty, this ridiculous caricature of the Paradise lost, only to be matched with Cotton's burlesque of Virgil, the illiterate herd of Booksellers paid the Translator one thousand pounds!'

37. TCD MS. 628. 2.26. According to Hill the French translator

> must ever fail in his attempts, because his Mind and Language are unpoetical; he is desperately ignorant of the Metaphors of English Poetry; and his crazed imagination, impetuously hurried on by Self-sufficiency and levity, will not pause to investigate and learn the Author's genuine sense; for which he hesitates not to substitute any thoughts, how remote soever from the truth, that may occur to his fancy, as they may happen to arise from a glimmering perception of the meaning of a word or two only in a period, whilst the context remains unintelligible.

38. TCD MS. 629. 4.85.

39. TCD MS. 629. 5.56.

40. TCD MS. 629. 5.34.

41. Charles Snyder (*Archives of Ophthalmology* [1963], 69: 531–3) has summarized the retrospective diagnoses offered for Milton's blindness:

> Punishment from the Almighty for Milton's role in the Cromwell Rebellion; gutta serena; cataract; albinism; neuroretinitis of congenital syphilitic origin; paralysis of the optic nerve; simple chronic glaucoma; due to a suprachiasmal cystic tumor which 'died' but destroyed his optic nerve in so doing; 'natural weakness'; complications of myopia; detachment of the retina; and acute glaucoma with attacks precipitated by emotional crises.

See also M. Dufour, 'Milton's Blindness', *The Ophthalmoscope* (1909), 7: 599–600; Arnold Sorsby, 'On the Nature of Milton's Blindness', *British Journal of Opthalmology* (1930), 1: 85–105; Eleanor G. Brown, *Milton's Blindness* (New York 1954); D. J. Wood, 'The Blindness of John Milton', *South African Medical Journal* (1935), 9: 791–5; L. R., *British Medical Journal* (1936), 2: 1275.

Modern eye specialists tend to favour either glaucoma or bilateral detached retina as the cause. A neurosurgeon, Lambert Rogers, suggested that the optic nerve fibres were destroyed by a cystic tumour pressing on the optic chiasma.

42. 'Erinensis' was the pseudonym of Dr Peter Hennis Green, who wrote for the *Lancet*.
43. Martin Fallon (ed.), *The Sketches of Erinensis* (London 1979), p. 138.
44. E.C. Nelson, 'Botany, Medicine and Politics in Eighteenth-Century Dublin', *Moorea* (1987), 6: 33–44.
45. William R. Parker, *Milton, A Biography*, vol. II (Oxford 1968), p. 1149.
46. E.J. Arnold, 'Edward Hill, M.D. (1741–1850) Editor of Milton', *Ann. Bull. Friends of the Library of Trinity College Dublin* (1951), 11–15.
47. TCD 10325/1–56 and 10326/1–34.
48. His daughter, Eliza, died in 1808. 'A few days illness deprived me of her in the end of last December, when she had survived her inestimable Mother, but a little more than one year.' TCD MS. 10326/11.
49. TCD MS. 10325/2.
50. TCD MS. 10325/5.
51. TCD MS. 10325/6.
52. TCD MS. 10325/7.
53. TCD MS. 10325/9.
54. TCD MS. 10325/10.
55. TCD MS. 10325/11.
56. TCD MS. 10325/12.
57. TCD MS. 10325/13.
58. Was this copy printed by Hill or was it a published edition corrected by him? It is unlikely to have been the interleaved copy. See note 82.
59. TCD MS. 10325/14.
60. TCD MS. 10325/16.
61. *Paradise Lost*, X, 661.
62. TCD MS. 10325/17.
63. TCD MS. 10325/18.
64. TCD MS. 10325/19.
65. TCD MS. 10325/20.
66. TCD MS. 10325/21.
67. TCD MS. 10325/24.
68. TCD MS. 10325/25.
69. TCD MS. 10325/26.
70. TCD MS. 10325/27.
71. TCD MS. 10325/28.
72. TCD MS. 10325/32.
73. Hill set out in the prospectus 36 examples of the errors in subsequent editions. A few examples given below cite book and line, the 1674 edition and the subsequent edition in that order. I, 673: was hid metallic ore / was hard metallic ore; III, 605: His native form / his naked form; IV, 708: Faunus haunted / Faunus hunted; V, 545: more delighted care / more delightful care; XII, 165: a sequent King; a frequent King.
    Collation of Hill's columns with the Oxford 'Standard Authors' rendering of *Paradise Lost* (Douglas Bush [ed.], *Milton Poetical Works* [London 1966]) shows that where Milton and Hill write 'Medal and

Stone (III, 592) the modern edition understandably prefers 'metal or stone'; the 1674 edition offers 'In shadie Bowre' (IV, 705) but the 1966 edition 'In shadier bower'. Hill defended 'shadie' in a lengthy note.

Referring to II, 730 – 'and know'st for whom;' – Hill complains in his Notes that Tickell incorrectly places a question mark after 'whom' instead of a semicolon. This 'error', if such it be, persists in the 1966 edition, which also includes 'Alablaster' (V, 544) altered by Hill to 'Alabaster', the spelling used in *Paradise Regained* – 'Alablaster is not warranted by any Lexicon or Dictionary whatsoever' (MS. 629/5/48).

According to Hill, 'the blanc Moon' (X, 656) is the pale moon denoted by the French term *blanc*; the 1966 Oxford edition reads 'the blank moon'.

74. TCD MS. 10325/46.
75. Arnold, *op. cit.*, p. 13.
76. On the subject of the School of Physic he wrote:

> I am not an Enemy to the School of Physic, but a zealous supporter of its real interests. But what can be denominated *a School of Physic*? Surely not a crowd of ill-taught School boys, and illiterate apprentices of Surgeons and Apothecaries, who, after having dozed for a stated period of time at the Lectures of Professors, find themselves privileged, on their producing a number of Certificates of their attendance, to apply for a Degree, without their understanding even the Alphabet of any of those Languages or Sciences, which are the indispensably-requisite preliminaries to a Profession the most difficult to learn . . .

RCPI MS. 14 Feb. 1812.

77. T.P.C. Kirkpatrick, *Edward Hill, M.D.* (Dublin 1920). Kirkpatrick refers unsympathetically to Hill's index as 'a monument of misdirected energy'.
78. *Ibid.*, p. 33. An undated letter from Hill (TCD MS. 10326/31) must refer to this or some other unhappy period when he was at odds with his colleagues:

> It has been my lot to entertain a friendship for and to place a confidence in several persons who were in all respects unworthy of my regard. Their hypocritical professions but disguised a disposition to injure me; And when an opportunity favor'd, they requited my kindness and numerous good offices with insult and ingratitude. Those apples on the Shores of the Asphaltic lake, whose golden rind allured the sight, whilst at the core lay dust and bitter ashes, are a proper type of them . . .

(*Paradise Lost*, X, 560–6)

79. His death passed unnoticed in the College minutes. His portrait was presented to the College of Physicians by his great-granddaughter, Miss Curtis, in 1914.
80. The Rev. William Hill was a skilled horologist and some lines were written in his honour by Mr Thomas O'Meara:

> There's a Naturalist called Parson Hill
> And in Mechanics who exceeds his skill [?]
> Good Clocks and Watches he can surely make
> Some at the Hours do make the Cuckoo speak . . .

81. Brennan's surgical degree was obtained in Glasgow and he was a Licentiate of the Apothecaries' Hall, Dublin. He practised at 80 Main Street, Carrick-on-Suir.

82. TCD MS. 10325/45. Hill had handed over to Brennan a manuscript in five volumes and two printed volumes. Were the latter the interleaved copies of *Paradise Lost* now in the library at TCD? Philip Dixon Hardy, the Dublin printer, mentioned to William Hill that he had in his possession, left with him by Edward Hill as a deposit against a debt for a small printing job, a volume of *Paradise Lost* collated with all the editions ever published. Was this the printed copy that Edward Hill sent to W.B. Taylor? See note 58.

83. TCD MS. 10325/46.

84. Bell, *op. cit.*, p. 255.

85. TCD MS. 10325/44. 'I got the within mentioned Books back from Brennan, on the 30th of August 1845, and paid him Ten Pounds for them in the presence of Alexander Vass.'

86. Edward Hill's other unpublished works include *A History of Medicine*, given by his nephew, Thomas Hill, to the RCSI, of which he was a licentiate, and *A Novell* [*sic*] – *Scythian Friendship* (TCD MS. 1015). His design for the Memorial to the Duke of Wellington, submitted in 1814, was rejected despite his claim that his memorial temple would continue to exist for a thousand years. His son made a model of the temple.

87. TCD MS. 10325/53. 'But as the work was a pet child of my grandfather he was unwilling to sell his rights in it for what was offered.'

4

Sir William Wilde, 1815–76

ON 1 April 1876 Sir William Wilde lay dying in his house in Merrion Square. His reputation at the time was under a cloud which later events in the Wildes' story did nothing to disperse. Dublin is quick to seize on the incongruous: Sir William and Speranza appeared to be an ill-suited pair – he was small, untidy and physically unprepossessing while she was tall and striking; his mind sought facts and their collation while hers was imaginative and fantastic. Wilde's white beard and dishevelled appearance led to puns on his name. 'Don't you know me?' he asked a fellow member of the British Association in 1874, 'I'm Wilde.' 'By God, you look it!' was the disconcerting response.[1] His notoriety was compounded by Lady Wilde's habit of overdressing and a love of gaudy jewellery, which made her seem like 'a walking mausoleum', and by her frequent parties in rooms shuttered against the daylight.[2] In his centenary year,* however, the extent of his interests and achievements seems remarkable and one looks to various authorities for verification of his competence in all. Primarily an ear and eye surgeon, and a statistician of professional attainments, his principal avocation was archaeology and he was awarded the Royal Irish Academy's Cunningham Medal, its highest award.

He was a great doctor and, according to T.G. Wilson, one of the two pioneers of ear surgery in the United Kingdom – the other was Joseph Toynbee, who, coincidentally, had a brilliant son, for whom Toynbee Hall was named.[3] Wilde's teachers would have been bewildered by a 'running' ear. Folk medicine held sway and remedies included plugging the ear with a sliver of fat

* Communication to a meeting in the RCSI on 1 April 1976; published in the *Journal of the Irish Colleges of Physicians and Surgeons* (1976), 5: 147–52.

bacon or with a wad of black wool, preferably wool taken from the left forefoot of a six-year-old black ram. When William Wilde's *Practical Observations on Aural Surgery* was published in 1853 his stated object was to equip ear surgery with scientific principles and to remove it from what he called 'that shroud of quackery, medical as well as popular, with which until lately it has been encompassed'.[4] Garrison and Morton's *Medical Bibliography* states: 'This work did more to place British otology on a sound scientific basis than anything previously published.'[5]

Colm Ó Lochlainn[6] ranked him with the leading Irish scientific archaeologists of his time and his catalogue of the Royal Irish Academy's collection of antiquities was a *tour de force*. Liam de Paor called it 'a milestone in the history of Irish archaeology', explaining that this 'was the first and last time that a full catalogue was produced of what subsequently became the core of the national collections of antiquities, now housed in the National Museum'.[7]

He was awarded a knighthood in 1864 for his work in connection with the Irish census and Sir Peter Froggatt made the following comment on the Census of Ireland 1851:

This was one of the greatest national censuses ever conducted. The results were published in ten foolscap volumes totalling 4,503 pages. Two of these volumes, containing 710 pages, were written solely by Wilde. The first, the 'States of Disease' contains the statistics on handicaps . . . the second, 'The Tables of Death', is one of the longest Blue Books ever written by one person. It contains, in addition to the customary analyses and report, over 300 pages in tabular format tracing the history of 'pestilences, cosmical phenomena, epizootics and famines', in Ireland from prehistoric period to 1850, with a full description of sources. This is a classic of great scholarship, erudition and industry, and is the standard reference work in the subject.[8]

The availability of such useful appraisals seems to make additional comment redundant. In a sense this is so: Wilde's contribution as editor of the *Dublin Quarterly Journal of Medical Science* and his topographical books have also received critical attention but the one aspect of his work lacking consideration as a whole is his scattered biographical output. Before dwelling on this it is appropriate to outline his career and allude to his own biographers.

VICTORIAN DOCTOR

The first major biography was T.G. Wilson's *Victorian Doctor* (1942); Patrick Byrne's *The Wildes of Merrion Square* followed in

1953; Eric Lambert's *Mad With Much Heart* and Terence de Vere White's *The Parents of Oscar Wilde* were both published in 1976. Byrne's book added nothing and its author adopted a novelist's licence to use his imagination. Lambert's production must be dismissed as an inaccurate and poorly written pot-boiler. De Vere White had access to unpublished letters which Wilson may not have had the time or the opportunity to consult and his book is valuable for that reason, but as Speranza outlived her husband by twenty years we are given rather more of her than of William. She emerges from behind the mask of eccentricity as a loving and indulgent mother, a loyal and courageous wife, never ignoble, never descending from her own high standard of behaviour.[9]

Wilson's *Victorian Doctor* remains the standard 'Life'. Its author had something of his subject's versatility – a talented artist, an ear, nose and throat surgeon and president of the Royal College of Surgeons in Ireland in 1958–60. His enhanced visual sense enabled him to present his readers with admirable pen-pictures such as that of William Wilde's father, a Roscommon general practitioner:

Thomas Wilde practised all his long life, and did his rounds on horseback until the end. He must have been worth seeing, when at nearly eighty years of age he cantered along on his spanking chestnut, encased in his voluminous, many-caped, riding-coat, broadbrimmed leather hat, buckskin smalls, top-boots, overalls, and spatter-dashes, with a red culgee coming up to the middle of his nose.[10]

William Wilde, the son of Dr Wilde and his wife, Emily Fynne, was born at Kilkeevin, near Castlerea, County Roscommon in 1815. His formal education was obtained at the Royal School, Banagher, the Diocesan School, Elphin, Dr Steevens's Hospital and the Park Street Medical School but no less important was the education he picked up in the company of a local poacher, Paddy Walsh, at the feet of Father Prendergast, the last Abbot of Cong, when he visited his mother's people in Ballymagibbon, and from a sportsman named Blake, to whom Wilde refers nostalgically in *Lough Corrib*:

Well, with all your faults, Dick Blake, I cannot but remember how well you taught me to ride, keeping my 'hands low down on the saddle' – what skilful directions for shooting, and training setters and pointers, you gave me; and with what pride you used to see me shoot the rising trout from off the bridge of Cross years ago.[11]

At the time that Wilde left Roscommon for Dublin he was, in Wilson's words, 'a dark ferrety-looking young man, below the average size, with retreating chin and a bright roving eye'. Physically he was unattractive but more than compensated in personality, energy and intellect. He took the Letters Testimonial of the RCSI on 13 March 1837 and because he had been unwell through overwork Dr Robert Graves recommended him as personal physician to a wealthy invalid who was going on a health cruise. This nine-month interlude between student-days and practice provided material for his first book, *The Narrative of a Voyage to Madeira, Teneriffe, and Along the Shores of the Mediterranean* (1839), which brought him £250, enabling him to go abroad to equip himself for the speciality he had decided to adopt, a decision influenced by the neglected eye diseases so evident in the dusty, sun-baked streets of Cairo and Alexandria during his visit to Egypt. About a year later, having sampled the practice of Moorfield's Hospital, London, and the Allegemine Krankenhaus, Vienna, he set up as an ear and eye surgeon at 15 Westland Row and converted an old stable into a dispensary for the poor. This was the forerunner of St Mark's Ophthalmic Hospital for Diseases of the Eye and Ear, which he established in Mark Street, off Great Brunswick Street, in 1844. Meanwhile in 1841 he had been appointed medical commissioner to the Irish census and was actively associated with all the other Irish censuses during his lifetime.

Growing affluent, Wilde moved to 21 Westland Row and on 12 November 1851 married Jane Francesca Elgee, a poet whose contributions to *The Nation* appeared over the pen-name 'Speranza'. Their children were William, Oscar, and Isola, who died in childhood. In Cameron's *History of the Royal College of Surgeons in Ireland*, published in 1886, we read, 'few names are more widely known than that of Mr Oscar Wilde'; in the second edition (1916) Cameron wrote, 'of his sad ending nothing need be said'.[12]

The further move to 1 Merrion Square symbolized Wilde's professional success. His holidays were spent in a fishing-lodge which he built on Illaunroe, a peninsula in Lough Fee in Connemara, and later in Moytura House near Cong. His avocations brought him in touch with many famous people. When Lord

Macaulay, who was then writing his *History*, came to inspect the
field of the Battle of the Boyne, Wilde, author of *The Beauties of
the Boyne* (1849), was his cicerone. His honours included the
Order of the Polar Star, bestowed by the King of Sweden,
honorary membership of the Antiquarian Society of Berlin, MD
honoris causa of Dublin University, and the knighthood conferred
in 1864.

Since this essay is by way of a centenary tribute it is not proposed to highlight the libel case in which Wilde's honour was
impugned, but it cannot be altogether omitted. Wilde's physical
nature included a strong vein of sexuality and though ugly and
somewhat unkempt he had a winning way with women. It was
an open secret that Dr Henry Wilson, Wilde's assistant, was his
natural son and he had other illegitimate children. The liaison that
led to litigation was with Miss Mary Josephine Travers, whom
William Stokes had referred to him when she was nineteen. She
was the daughter of Dr Robert Travers, professor of medical
jurisprudence in TCD, whom T.G. Wilson dismisses, perhaps
unfairly, as 'an insignificant woolly-minded creature', for the
present Keeper of Archbishop Marsh's Library, where for years
Travers was assistant librarian, says he was a splendid scholar who
had 'contributed extensively to distinguished literary journals'.[13]

Wilde developed an affection for Mary Josephine which
initially may have been innocent and fatherly but there can be
little doubt that eventually the relationship exceeded the bounds
of propriety. Perhaps it was Wilde's decision (or Speranza's) that
the affair must end which caused a rift in their friendship. In any
event, Miss Travers, by then unbalanced, became his persecutor;
she published scurrilous doggerel in the press and circulated
offensive pamphlets. The time came when Lady Wilde, unable
to stand it any longer, penned a letter to the young woman's
father which contained statements that could be interpreted as
libellous.

The letter fell into the hands of the jilted lover, who sued
Lady Wilde for libel, her real motive in bringing the action being
the opportunity to cast obloquy on Sir William's reputation. In
court she accused him of having raped her in his surgery. That
charge was pooh-poohed by the judge but she won the libel
action and was awarded a farthing damages.

Because Lady Wilde was the actual defendant, Sir William was not obliged to give evidence. Wisely, he avoided appearing as a witness and for this he was castigated in the *Dublin Medical Press*, founded by his rival and enemy, Arthur Jacob, and edited at the time by the latter's son, Archibald, who maintained that Wilde should have denied his patient's allegations: 'He owed it to his profession which must now endure the onus of the disgrace – he owed it to the public, who have confided themselves to his honour – he owed it to Her Majesty's Representative, who had conferred an unusual mark of distinction on him, to purge himself of the suspicion which at this moment lies heavy on his name.'[14]

In the peace and quiet of Moytura House, Sir William allowed the scandal to subside and began to write what was to be his most popular book, *Lough Corrib, Its Shores and Islands* (1867).

SIR THOMAS MOLYNEUX

Turning now to the biographical output, the first offering was a long article on Sir Thomas Molyneux, written when Wilde was attending Moorfields Hospital. It was published in 1841 in the *Dublin University Magazine*, which also contains Wilde's articles on Sir Henry Marsh, Robert Graves and Sir Robert Kane. While editing the *Dublin Quarterly Journal of Medical Science* between 1845 and 1849 he introduced a series on illustrious Irish physicians and surgeons. An enquiry from a colleague in Glasgow in 1846 directed his attention to Jonathan Swift and resulted in a book called *The Closing Years of Dean Swift's Life*. His article on Dr Richard Steevens appeared in the *Medical Times and Gazette* (1856). His *Memoir of Gabriel Beranger* was published serially in the early 1870s in the *Journal of the Royal Archaeological Association of Ireland*.

A characteristic feature of Wilde's biographical essays is discursiveness; he lacked the true instinct of a biographer, being less interested in the man than in his achievements. He pursued his task with his usual capacity for collecting facts but had no gift for their deployment. 'It is the personal, Sir, that interests mankind,' said Dr Johnson to Boswell but Wilde overlooks this or perhaps that kind of information was lacking.

Most of Wilde's subjects were men of his own stamp with multiple interests and accomplishments in diverse fields. The 77-page essay on Sir Thomas Molyneux, the first Irish medical baronet, is one of Wilde's best biographies and drew on unpublished letters of Sir Thomas and his brother, William, one of the founders of the Dublin Philosophical Society and author of *The Case of Ireland Stated*, which was burned by the common hangman.[15]

He introduced the Molyneuxes, an Anglo-Norman family, with a coruscating metaphor:

A brief notice of this family, from their first settlement in Ireland, to the death of Sir Thomas, will carry us down a stream of time, broken by the boiling surge of civil wars, reversal of dynasties, and national degradation; and dashing headlong, like some mountain torrent from rock to rock – upturning, in its course, the barriers of social order, and swamping the flowery fields of literary and scientific knowledge, until, mingling with the calm and placid waters of more quiet and civilized times, it will hurry us through the history of events long since passed; and we trust for ever.[16]

The second son of Captain Samuel ('Honest Sam') Molyneux, a skilled mathematician and master gunner of Ireland, and his wife, Margaret Dowdall, Thomas Molyneux was born in Dublin on 14 April 1661 in his father's house near Ormond-gate. Educated in Dr Henry Rider's school and Dublin University he graduated MA and MB (1683) and, determined to enlarge his horizons, arrived in London on 15 May 1683.

He 'took up lodgings at the sign of the Flower-de-Luce, over against St Dunstan's Church in Fleet-street'[17] and when writing to his brother described the notabilities he met at Gresham College:

Mr Flamsteed I take to be a free, affable, and humble man, not at all conceited or dogmatical . . . I was but a short time in Mr Boyle's company, and therefore am not fit to give you any sort of character of him. He stutters, though not much; speaks very slow with many circumlocutions, just as he writes . . . Mr Hook . . . I am told that he is the most ill-natured, self-conceited man in the world, hated and despised by most of the Royal Society. Dr Grew is of a very unhealthy complexion, speaks mighty slow, and I believe has some disease in his lung. I am told he is no very profound physican.[18]

He also met John Dryden, the poet, and called on Elias Ashmole 'at his house beyond Lambeth'. The latter's collection went to form the nucleus of the Ashmolean Museum in Oxford.

Having spent some days there, Molyneux sent his brother a minute account of Cambridge. 'The vice-chancellor never allows more than 4 taverns in the town, and it is in his power to make them sell their wine at what rates he pleases.'[19] He went next to Oxford but, as the colleges were so well described in books which William had already read, he devoted his letter to an account of the masters and others. He had heard the professor of medicine, Dr Luff, 'read on the first aphorism of Hippocrates [*Ars longa, vita brevis* . . .] in the physic school . . .'[20] and discuss the shortness of man's life since the flood and its length before that event. 'I lodged in Oxford over against the theatre, at one Mrs Momphort's, a very old woman; she remembers Dorothea Wadham, one of the founders of Wadham College.'[21]

He sailed in July from Gravesend to Rotterdam, where he was impressed by the cathedral and the bronze statue of Erasmus. He proceeded to Leyden but before settling there visited Amsterdam, Harlem and Utrecht.

In Leyden he resided 'at the widow Vander-Stein's in the Long Bridge-street' and noticed 'that haulting, wadling, and limping men and women and children were extraordinary frequent and common'. The Dutch women's broad, misshapen feet he attributed to their inveterate habit of wearing loose slippers. Despite the reported absence of beggars in Holland he encountered them in Amsterdam and elsewhere.[22]

Fresh from his own *wanderjahr*, Wilde relished Molyneux's excitement in arranging private teaching from selected teachers, including Dr Margrave, 'an old experienced physician, a high German, that is allowed by the curators, though he be not a professor, to take private colleges'. Eventually he lived at Margrave's in order to have the advantage of his company and ready advice, and

also the uses of his glasses and furnaces whenever I shall have a mind to do any thing in chymistry myself . . . Here I shall have the advantage of speaking nothing but Lattin; and, moreover, I shall have the company of one or two friends, students in physic, very ingenious men, now living in this house . . . [23]

William Molyneux, meanwhile, had described for his brother the founding of the Dublin Philosophical Society.

I have also here promoted the rudiments of a society for which I have drawn up rules, and called it *Conventio Philosophica*. About half a score or a dozen of us have met about twelve or fifteen times, and we have very regular discourses concerning philosophical, medical, and mathematical matters.[24]

The winter of 1683–4 was bitterly cold in Holland. A soldier died on sentry duty at the Hague and two or three homeless children died of hunger and cold in Leyden. Dublin fared likewise and William Molyneux confirmed that the Liffey was frozen over for six weeks. He also referred to the recently completed Royal Hospital: "tis a most stately beautiful piece of building perhaps as Christendom affords for that use".[25]

William urged his brother to observe laboratories closely so that on his return 'we shall be the erecters and massers of as good a laboratory as can be desired for all chymical and astronomical operations, together with a convenient place for dissection . . .'.[26] Thomas visited Huygens at the Hague and was shown many instruments, including one resembling a clock. 'This shows you at once the minute, hour, day of the month and year, with the exact postures and aspects that all the planets bear to the sun and one another at that very moment . . .'.[27]

In August 1684 his first article, which concerned 'the dissolution and swimming of heavy bodies in Menstruums far lighter than themselves', was published in *Nouvelles de la République des Lettres* and in December he sent his first contribution to the *Philosophical Transactions*, an account of a 'prodigious *os frontis*'. While in Leyden he compiled a catalogue for the Royal Society of the zoological collections of Swammerdam and Herman. In 1685 he spent some time in Paris, accompanied temporarily by his brother. He visited the more important libraries but was disappointed by the hospitals. In the following year he was elected FRS.

On his return to Dublin in April 1687 he took the MD and set up in practice but because of the unsettled state of the country he left Ireland towards the end of 1688 and for a time practised in Chester. After William of Orange's victory at the Boyne he returned to Dublin and resumed practice with immediate success. He published an essay on renal stones in the *Philosophical Transactions* in 1693.

The previous year had seen the death of his father and the election of William Molyneux as university representative in the Irish parliament. Thomas married in 1693; his bride was Catherine Howard, a daughter of Dr Robert Howard of Shelton, County Wicklow, a woman of considerable beauty and character. They were to have sixteen children, of whom four did not survive infancy.

William Molyneux died on 11 October 1698 from a severe haematemesis at the early age of forty-two. Among the letters of sympathy which Thomas received was one from John Locke, whom he first met in Leyden and had been in correspondence with as medical adviser for some years.

Molyneux was president of the College of Physicians for three terms and held important public offices – state physician, physician general to the army, professor of the practice of medicine in Dublin University. He amassed a fortune from his extensive practice and built a mansion in Peter Street, which he furnished lavishly. When somebody ventured to compare his fortune with that of Dr Steevens he boasted that he had *spent* more than Steevens ever earned.

He was fortunate in his marriage and despite her large family his artistic wife found time to adorn his mansion with her own paintings. And she could use her pencil, Wilde tells us, 'to more advantage than mere amusement; for she drew the originals of all the engravings published in the different writings of her husband'.[28] These provided the material for the concluding section of Wilde's biography. They included articles on the extinct Irish elk, the Irish wolf dog, Horace's odes and the ancient Greek and Roman lyre.

The confidential nature of medical practice generally places a doctor's day-to-day activities at a remove from his biographer but in any case Wilde may have preferred to deal with Molyneux's avocations, which appealed to his own encyclopedic mind. In 'A Discourse concerning the Danish Mounts, Forts and Towers in Ireland' Molyneux refuted a prevalent belief that the existence of cinerary urns in ancient burial places was an indication of a Roman conquest of Ireland.

Wilde felt that 'Some Observations on the Taxes paid by Ireland to support the Government', an unpublished manuscript written in 1727, reveals Molyneux, who died in 1733, as something of a statesman and political economist. 'He was for forty years the leading physician in Ireland; and it was not without good reason that John Locke chose him as his friend and adviser.'[29]

The author acknowledged his debt to General Sir Thomas Molyneux, Bart, 'for his liberal contribution of family documents'. James Hardiman also helped him but Wilde relegated Molyneux's journey to Galway in 1709 to a footnote, thus losing the opportunity to highlight the physician's visit to Roderic O'Flaherty, the historian, in Connemara. Shared interests facilitate warm relationships but one wonders if during their conversation on that April afternoon in the octogenarian's wind-swept house either man was struck by how aptly they personified the Irish and the Anglo-Irish strains.

SIR HENRY MARSH, BART

Wilde envied biographers who dealt with statesmen and heroes, whose careers abound in attractive incidents sufficient to kindle readers' interest. 'How shall the career and merits of the physician be rendered interesting by detail?' he asked. 'His studies are performed, and his exploits achieved in a science whose very terms are unintelligible to the uninitiated, and whose principles are not understood even by the learned.' And while the maxim *de mortuis nil nisi bonum* merited respect he believed 'that praise of the living is fulsome'.[30]

Henry Marsh was born to the manse at Loughrea, County Galway in 1790. He was the scion of a family that flourished in Gloucestershire, the first to settle in Ireland being his great-grandfather, Archbishop Francis Marsh, who married Mary, daughter of Jeremy Taylor, the celebrated Bishop of Down and Connor and sometime chaplain to Charles I, who on the day before his execution gave him his watch. (This, Wilde noted with antiquarian zeal, was 'a large gold watch in a pinch beck case'; it remained a treasured possession in the elder branch of Sir Henry Marsh's family and continued to keep excellent time.) His parents were the Rev. Robert Marsh, rector of Killinane, and his wife, Sophia, daughter of the Rev. William Wolseley, rector of Tullycorbet, County Monaghan.

He lost his mother in the first year of his life and at a tender age attended a classical school in Loughrea which Wilde tells us was 'as famous at that time for the severity of its discipline as for the number of celebrated scholars it produced'.[31]

Scholarship was not, however, the Rev. Marsh's objective for he encouraged his son to work on the glebe farm until a chance encounter with a stranger who happened to know his uncle, the Rev. Digby Marsh FTCD, turned the lad's mind to other pursuits and to the rewards of learning.

He took the BA at TCD in 1812 and again preferred to make his own choice of career, opting to be a surgeon rather than please his father by becoming a clergyman. He planned to take advantage of the demand for surgeon's-mates in the Peninsula but was persuaded instead to be apprenticed to his cousin, Philip Crampton, at the Meath Hospital. Having accepted the uncongenial alternative as safer though less adventurous he sustained a wound while dissecting and lost the index finger of his right hand. A career in surgery being now closed to him, he switched to medicine. He spent a year in Paris at La Charité and on his return to Dublin, skilled in the use of the stethoscope, was appointed assistant to his cousin, John Crampton, physician to Dr Steevens's Hospital.

If the ingredients of success in medicine are 'the three A's' ability, availability and affability, Marsh must have possessed them in ample measure for before long he was spectacularly successful. He held a chair in medicine at the College of Surgeons (1887–32); he was appointed physician in ordinary to the Queen in Ireland (1837) and created a baronet (1839).

Wilde credited Sir Henry Marsh with possessing a 'rare gift of penetrating observation . . . and an almost unerring judgement'. Observation, he believed, was the essential quality.

Observation, guided by reason, prudence, and judgement, we believe to be the genius of all consummate intellectual attainment, whether general or professional; – like poetry it is a gift at birth, and is not in the endowment of art; it must be *brought* to the academy, it is not to be *found there*; it belongs to the individual, and is a part of the man, who will manifest it in his vocation, be it whatever it may be. In all professions, it is a *sine qua non* of absolute perfection; but in medicine, it is in practical requisition at every stage of every case. Destitute of this qualification, the physician, however well educated, however scientific, seldom rises to eminence; he may practise creditably, nay, usefully, but he possesses not the *talisman* of his art.[32]

Wilde also acknowledged Sir Henry's 'urbanity and honourable deportment towards his juniors'. He presented a 'sketch' or profile rather than a biography.

ROBERT GRAVES

When Robert Graves (honoured still by the eponym 'Graves's disease') agreed to appear in the *Dublin University Magazine*'s

'Portrait Gallery' he asked that Wilde, his 'friend and pupil', should write the memoir.[33] Wilde accepted the commission on the understanding that only he and the editor should see the article prior to publication. He knew that 'portraits' had been tampered with by zealous friends.

Graves supplied him with a sheet of foolscap bearing dates and certain facts to be included but discouraged the broader representation that might have been attempted. When, for instance, Wilde sought to verify the date of a celebrated incident in which Graves had taken command of a sinking ship in the Mediterranean and, by using shoe-leather to mend the pumps, averted a catastrophe, the physician said: 'Don't mind any of these things; don't say anything about the little tailor and the crazy ship. It is true I saved my life on that occasion but all I want now is to save the lives of others, especially of good Irishmen . . .'.[34] A further constraint was imposed by the undesirability of repeating facts about the Graves family given in the periodical by the Rev. R.H. Graves two years previously in a review of the *Works of Dean Graves*.

A pen-and-ink sketch was supplied by Charles Gray RHA, but Wilde felt it lacked 'the searching gaze, the animated expression, and bright piercing eye, which no illustration can ever portray'. Dr and Mrs Graves thought the article, on its appearance on 1 February 1842, to be 'fair and judicious'. The author republished it as a booklet in 1864 but even then he did not take advantage of the removal of earlier constraints and provide a substantial biography.[35] What he did achieve was an account of Graves the educationalist seen through the eyes of a younger contemporary. Within those limitations he makes a unique contribution: he conveys the students' excitement in the extended universe revealed by the microscope and their new-found interest in current research. He tells how they turned up in large numbers to hear Graves lecture at four o'clock:

Then all weariness was forgotten, all langour vanished; the note books were again resumed – the attention that had already flagged at an early hour of the day was aroused by the absorbing interest of the subject, and the energy of the lecturer; nay more, the noisy bustle usually attendant on the breaking up of a lecture was exchanged for discussions upon the subjects treated on, or eager inquiries of the Professor for the solution of difficulties, and the freshness of morning again came over the exhausted student's mind.[36]

Recalling his own arduous studies and conscious, no doubt, of the collective defamation of medical students by Charles Dickens in the *Pickwick Papers* where Bob Sawyer is depicted as looking 'something like a dissipated Robinson Crusoe' with an inordinate interest in brandy and oysters, Wilde undertook their defence:

The public, and we regret to add the public press, have of late years been pleased to consider that portion of the community yclept medical students as being beyond the pale of human sympathies – creatures who, by the very name they bear, have become unfit associates for the rich and good, barely worthy of acknowledgment by their own connexions, fair game at which to hurl every description of missile, from the satire of a 'saw-bones' to the merciless abuse of a morning paper. How few ever consider the peculiar position in which one of those young gentlemen is suddenly placed, who arrives, perhaps for the first time in his life, in the metropolis, from beneath the paternal roof![37]

The student rises early to visit the hospital; he attends lectures endlessly and runs from them to the dissecting-room or the chemist's laboratory; he is exposed hourly to infectious maladies and other dangers. The system of education – or the lack of system – was lamentable. Graves, 'the first great medical teacher we have had in this country', had improved the situation by introducing despite opposition and ridicule the system favoured in Germany.

Robert James Graves, the youngest son of Richard Graves DD (commonly called 'Pentateuch' Graves in recognition of his biblical studies), and his wife, Eliza (*née* Drought), was born in Holles Street, Dublin, on 28 March 1796. His father became professor of divinity and Dean of Ardagh, by which time Robert had entered TCD, where he read a brilliant course in arts and medicine, graduating BA (1815) and MB (1818). His postgraduate teachers in London included Sir William Blizzard, an acquaintance of Oliver Goldsmith, and he spent two years in Berlin, visiting also medical centres in Göttingen, Copenhagen, France and Italy. He returned to Ireland in 1821 and his appointment to the Meath Hospital, though queried by the board of governors,[38] enabled him to introduce basic educational changes.

One of the founders of the Park Street School of Medicine, he applied successfully for the professorship of the institutes of medicine in 1827 and was co-editor of the *Dublin Journal of Medical Science*. Under his new scheme at the Meath Hospital students studied disease, as Wilde explains, 'not from the well-devised oration . . . but by observing all its forms, changes and symptoms at the bedside; by having patients submitted to his care, under the direction of the physician . . .'.

Wilde's terms of reference did not permit him to tell his readers anything of his subject's home life (Graves had a socially conscious wife, whose dinner guests at 84 Merrion Square included the viceroy) in Dublin or at Cloghan Castle near Banagher, which he bought to placate Mrs Graves's ambition to rank among the gentry. The closest the author comes to revealing something of Graves's character in his maturity is the statement that he 'combines in a remarkable degree, decision and candour – the latter, perhaps, even to a fault – '.[39]

Andrew Young, a 'dresser' in the old Meath Hospital, recalled Graves as a 'lithe, dark-haired, eagle-eyed, and energetic mannered gentleman',[40] but his portrait in maturity reveals the tight-lipped, turned-down mouth of a depressed countenance. Sir Charles Cameron remarked that Graves's practice declined 'not because he was becoming too old (for he died in the prime of life) but for some reasons difficult to understand'.[41] Wilde shed no light on the mystery nor did he allude to it. Graves died on 20 March 1853.

SIR ROBERT KANE

After two closely printed pages of generalizations and reflections on 'this every-day-working world of ours, progressing as it is with railroad speed', Wilde at last offers biographical data: born in Dublin in 1810, Robert Kane was educated for the medical profession, 'His early tendency to chemical pursuits, probably arose from his family having been chemical manufacturers in this city.'[42]

A list of the disastrous consequences and collapse resulting from the Union is then introduced. But the school of medicine was the first among Irish institutions 'to raise itself from this thraldom and inactivity' and young Kane was fortunate in his teachers, Graves and Stokes, at the Meath Hospital, where in 1830 he was awarded a prize for an essay on the 'Pathological Condition of the Fluids in Typhus Fever.'[43]

While still a student, Kane was appointed professor of chemistry at the Apothecaries' Hall, then an important educational body, and held the post until 1845. He published *The Elements of Practical Pharmacy* (1831) and founded the *Dublin Journal of Medical and Chemical Science* (1832). In 1838 he married Katherine Baily, author of *The Irish Flora* (1833) and niece to Francis Baily, the astronomer. He was elected Fellow of the King and Queen's College of Physicians of Ireland (the present RCPI) in 1841 but, understandably, Wilde did not mention directly Kane's early difficulties with the College of Physicians.

When Kane wished to sit for the Licentiateship of the College of Physicians in 1833 it was moved by the vice-president, Dr James Henry, and seconded by Dr Robert Law, 'that Mr Kane being a Licentiate Apothecary and Director of the Apothecaries' Hall his admission as Licentiate of the College of Physicians is inconsistent with the 5th By Law in chapter 5'.[44] Henry's resolution was passed by eight votes to one. Kane reapplied for examination, explaining that just then he could not resign his position as director of the Hall but James Henry insisted on the letter of the law and not until 1835 was Kane accepted as a candidate, having submitted written proof that he was no longer a director. He passed the examination in May 1835. Four years later he was proposed and seconded for election to Fellowship but the proposal was withdrawn without explanation in October and resubmitted in October 1840. On the occasion of that election, Kane, a chemist and a Catholic, was rejected when the tally showed four white beans and five black ones.[45]

Wilde provides a step-by-step account of the evolution of Kane's career and achievements – his election as MRIA and his work as secretary to the council; his chair of natural philosophy at the RDS, 1834–47, and his course of lectures on the sources of industry which exist in Ireland; the researches on ammoniacal compounds of mercury, copper and zinc for which he was awarded the RIA's Cunningham medal; the work on the colouring matters of lichens which gained for him the Royal Society's royal medal: his directorship of the Museum of Irish Industry in St Stephen's Green. His publications included *The Elements of Chemistry* (1841–2), which Michael Faraday used for his classes at Woolwich, and *The Industrial Resources of Ireland*, which went into a second edition within months of its first appearance in 1844. Two years later Kane was honoured by the honorary membership of the RDS, a knighthood and his appointment as first president of Queen's College, Cork.

Reflecting that the premises of the Museum of Irish Industry was the former town house of Lord Chancellor Manners, Wilde digressed sharply to list the fate of many fine houses – Belvedere House a school, Moira House a shelter for mendicants, the former stamp-office, Powerscourt House, 'now filled with linsey-woolseys and Manchester cottons' – and ventured to speculate on what might happen to others.

In a few years more, if the present system of centralisation is carried out, we suppose we shall see Dublin Castle a head police-office; the Four Courts will probably be converted into a city marshalsea or an additional poorhouse; the viceregal residence at the Phoenix-park a model farm; the Richmond Hospital a convict depot, and the Royal Hospital at Kilmainham, a refuge for decayed detectives.[46]

He concluded his biographical essay with a fine paragraph of forceful prose which placed Kane before his readers as a model worthy of imitation:

To the slothful and the indolent, wasting their time in vain repinings for the unhappy position either of their own affairs or the condition of the country generally – to the sneering and captious, who try to discover for other men's rewards and greatness some unworthy reason – to the vapouring politician, who wastes his own time and that of others in useless agitation – to the young and unknown aspirant after fame, who fears there may be no room for him in the crowded halls of science; – to every Irishman who will calmly examine the course which Sir Robert Kane has trodden; who will review his past career; struggling with difficulties – difficulties of position, of fortune, and, at one time, of religion – his vigorous dynamical intellect and fierce energy, bursting the thraldom in which accident had bound him – snatching the highest rewards which science holds out to her votaries – elevating the land in which we live, by associating himself with her truest and best interests, and spreading abroad her fame upon the pages of literature and science – earning for the present the title of patriot, and carving for himself a name which history shall transmit to future time – to all, we would say: the road is open, go and do likewise.[47]

ILLUSTRIOUS IRISH PHYSICIANS AND SURGEONS

Six articles appeared under this heading in the *Dublin Quarterly Journal of Medical Science* during Wilde's editorship. Those on Sir Patrick Dun and David McBride were by Aquilla Smith; that on John Rutty, the liveliest of the lot, was by Jonathan Osborne, and Wilde contributed biographies of Bartholomew Mosse, John Oliver Curran and Sylvester O'Halloran. The essay on Mosse contains long extracts from a manuscript by Benjamin Higgins, clerk to the Lying-in Hospital, or, as we call it nowadays, the Rotunda Hospital, outlining its development, the granting of a charter and the appointment of the first Master. It is well that this material should be preserved but it does not make for good biography. Wilde's generous quotations from a correspondence between Mosse and Giovanni Battista Cipriani, an Italian artist working in England, were also fortunate for the original letters are lost.[48]

Bartholomew Mosse, the second son of the Rev. Thomas Mosse, rector of Maryborough (now Portlaoise), was born in 1712 and apprenticed to John Stone, a Dublin surgeon, being certified competent to practise in 1733. Having supervised the transport of troops to Minorca he travelled in England and continental Europe and on his return to Dublin conceived the ambition of providing the city with an amenity not then available in any English-speaking country, a lying-in hospital. This opened in George's Lane on 15 March 1745 – its first patient, Judith Rochford, was delivered of a son five days later. In 1748 he leased a piece of ground in Great Britain Street, where the New Garden was soon established and the building, erected to the design of Richard Cassells (or Castle), was opened on 8 December 1757.

'The doctor was, at the time of opening the hospital [in George's Lane], about thirty-three years of age, in full health and vigour, of a clear understanding, affable and agreeable in his conversation and behaviour . . .'.[49] Despite a pleasing personality and a praiseworthy purpose, traducers circulated reports to his disadvantage; it was rumoured 'that he had taken the lease in his own name, and for the use of himself and his family without any intention of building a hospital; and that, under the specious pretence of public charity he was then exhorting large sums of money with which he meant to quit the kingdom'.[50] He countered this accusation by setting up a trust which was duly registered and he obtained a charter in 1755.

Mosse planned to have the hospital chapel sumptuously decorated. When Cipriani was engaged to execute the paintings in the ceiling Mosse cautioned him that as the chapel was intended for Protestant worship only, 'I would have the painting entirely free from any superstitious or Popish representation.'[51] Whereupon Cipriani assured him, tongue in cheek, 'that you shall have no other Popery in the picture than the Nativity of our Saviour; and, as I am pretty sure that the Pope shall never set foot in Ireland, so you may be confident that my picture will never contribute to the enlargement of His Holiness's jurisdiction.'[52]

Within a year of the consummation of his ambition Mosse's health failed and his life ended on 16 February 1759. He 'died poor as to wealth, but rich in the blessings of the needy'.[53] His great creation, which, after the completion of John Ensor's round room in 1767, was called the Rotunda Hospital, was to attain international prominence but in due course the Rev. Richard Graves DD rebuked the Rotunda from the pulpit for permitting drunkenness and debauchery in its assembly rooms and garden. 'Gracious God!' the cleric protested, 'what are we to say to this? What a satire it is on the nation to suppose that no means can be found to supply the funds of such a charity, but by corrupting public morals, and patronising the violation of the Sabbath of the Lord!'

The account of Dr John Oliver Curran,[54] a typhus victim, opens with Wilde's irrefutable statement about the famine.

The present year is now drawing to a close; and all who have witnessed its singular and melancholy scenes must look back upon it with wonder and with dread. Its history will be a darkened age in the annals of our country, recording events whose nature may warrant the incredulity of after times. It will be difficult to believe at a future, and we hope, a happier day, that, within a short distance of the capital of England, the seat of British intelligence, British power, wealth and plenty, nearly a million of her subjects died of hunger or its consequences; of want, not resulting from their own improvidence, but from the long-threatened, yet not till then complete failure of a crop which was their only support. The record of this great and dreadful fact is engraved in characters so deep and strong that ages will not efface them.[55]

Curran was born at Troopersfield, near Lisburn, in 1819 and reared in the Isle of Man before entering the universities of Glasgow and Dublin. He took the MB of the latter in 1843 and spent a post-graduate year in Paris prior to his appointment as honorary physician to the Dublin General Dispensary and professor of the practice of medicine to the Apothecaries' Hall.

When an epidemic necessitated the erection of fever-sheds at Kilmainham and elsewhere in 1847 the Board of Health set about recruiting a staff of medical officers. Curran offered his services promptly and was appointed but resigned on learning that he was to be paid five shillings a day, pointing out that such remuneration was not consistent with the dignity and honour of his profession.

This protest did not place him beyond the perils of infection; he gave his time and skill without charge to the dispensary patients and when two French medical commissioners arrived to observe the epidemic he conducted them to the various institutions. Then M. Gueneau de Mussy, one of the French doctors, fell ill with fever and Curran acted as his nurse, seldom leaving him, day or night, until he too sickened, a fatal victim of what Wilde called 'the Moloch of pestilence'.[56]

The last article in this series was on Sylvester O'Halloran,[57] who had shared Wilde's interest in opthalmology and his passion for Irish antiquities; its prolixity is lightened by the inclusion of Dr Charles Kidd's recollections of the Limerick surgeon, who, incidentally, may have been the model for Count O'Halloran, a character in Maria Edgeworth's novel *The Absentee*.[58]

JONATHAN SWIFT

The importance of Wilde's work on Swift is that he was the first to refute the popular supposition that the great satirist was 'mad':

neither in his expressions, nor the tone of his writing, nor from an examination of any of his acts, have we been able to discover a single symptom of insanity, nor aught but the effects of physical disease, and the natural wearing and decay of a mind such as Swift's.

The study was prompted by a request from a Glasgow oculist, Dr W. Mackenzie, that Swift's health problems should be reviewed in the *Dublin Quarterly Journal of Medical Science*. Wilde complied with a long article, 'Some Particulars respecting Swift and Stella'.[59] This was followed by *The Closing Years of Dean Swift's Life* (1849), a fascinating book rich in details of the Dean's ailments. As an ear surgeon, Wilde was puzzled by Swift's deafness and vertigo, which he attributed to 'cerebral congestion', a rather vague concept. Nowadays Swift is thought to have suffered from Ménière's disease.[60]

Recalling that the remains of Swift and Stella were exhumed during repairs to the cathedral in 1835, Wilde described vividly how Swift's skull was carried unceremoniously from hall to hall at the British Association's Dublin meeting.

The University, where Swift had so often toiled again beheld him, but in another phase; the Cathedral which heard his preaching, – the Chapter-house which echoed his sarcasm, – the Deanery which resounded with his sparkling wit, and where he gossiped with Sheridan and Delany, – the lanes and alleys which knew his charity, the squares and streets where the people shouted his name in the days of his unexampled popularity, – the mansions where he was the honoured and much-sought guest, – perhaps the very rooms he often visited were again occupied by the dust of Swift.[61]

Admiring an engraving of Stella's skull, Wilde called it 'a perfect model of symmetry and beauty':

On the whole, it is no great stretch of the imagination to clothe and decorate this skull again with its alabaster skin, on which the rose had slightly bloomed; to adorn it with its original luxuriant dark-brown hair, its white expanding forehead, level pencilled eye-brows, and deep lustrous eyes, its high Roman nose, its delicately chiselled mouth, its short pouting upper lip, its full rounded chin, and graceful swelling neck . . . .[62]

Wilde derided a votary of phrenology who, having measured the Dean's exhumed skull, reported 'small intellectual and large animal propensities – Little wit and great amativeness – '.[63]

T.G. Wilson accused Wilde of making 'the most unwarranted assumptions and conclusions' but, nevertheless, he regarded *The Closing Years of Dean Swift's Life* as an important book.[64]

DR RICHARD STEEVENS

Wilde's account of Richard Steevens and his hospital suffered the handicap imposed by the lack of material. He offers all that is known of Steevens: the son of the rector of Athlone, an Englishman driven out by Cromwell, he was intended for the Church but switched to medicine and became wealthy without holding public office or attaining any acclaim for professional publications; he was unmarried and would willingly have left his fortune to Griselda, his twin sister, but as it was apparent that she, too, would remain celibate, he devised it to her on his death for her lifetime and after her decease to establish a hospital for the sick poor.[65]

Madame Steevens was something of a recluse to which habit Wilde attributed the legend that she had a face like a pig. This nasty story persisted despite the existence of her portrait, which, as he pointed out, 'beams with comeliness, intelligence and benevolence'.[66] He recalled paying a penny as a lad to look into a 'peep-show' which depicted her deformed image eating out of a silver trough. The kindly lady decided that Dublin's poor should not have to wait until her death to enjoy her civic-minded brother's plans for their welfare. She reserved £150 per annum her own use and an apartment in the new hospital, which was built without further delay. Dr Steevens's Hospital opened in 1733. It notable benefactors included Hester Johnson (Swift's 'Stella') who endowed a chaplaincy, and Dr Edward Worth, who presented his magnificent library to the hospital.

Wilde retained a natural affection for his teaching-hospital and described it as he and Charles Lever, the novelist, would have known it in the mid-1830s:

Twenty years ago there resided in Steevens' Hospital about thirty pupils . . . These young men were of all grades of studentship, from the entered apprentice to the man going in for his degree; they lived anywhere and everywhere, in pupils rooms, and in holes and corners, as they could be best stowed away. Possibly the majority were idle; yet they learned, and that, too, by a mode not within the pupil's reach now. Steevens' Hospital was then the favourite of the Dublin public, and the great resort of accidents and operations; thus the accident bell rang, upon an average, every two hours, day and night; and upon each occasion the whole class, idle or industrious, rushed to the reception room. There they saw – not as pupils now see Cases 'done up' and in bed on the morning visit of the Surgeon with whom they 'walk' the Hospital but in all their original freshness, compound fractures, severed throats, ruptured perinaeums, extensive burns, injuries of the head, recent poisonings, lacerated wounds, crushed limbs, and, in the course of a few months, all the routine of Surgical practice.[67]

Tents were erected in the hospital's laundry-yard during fever epidemics; at other times it served as a military hospital and a Lock Hospital. In the present century, prior to its unexpected closure in the late 1980s, it housed departments of orthopaedic and plastic surgery and a burns unit, while the unique Worth Library was a particular treasure.

GABRIEL BERANGER*

Gabriel Beranger, a Huguenot artist and antiquarian with a print-shop in South Georges Street, came to Dublin from Rotterdam in 1750. He married his cousin, Miss Beranger, and later a Mademoiselle Mestayer. He died without issue in 12 St Stephen's Green south in his eighty-ninth year and was buried in the French cemetery in Peter Street. During his life he made a number of tours in Ireland and his description of these makes up the bulk of Wilde's book.

The serial publication of the *Memoir of Gabriel Beranger* began in the *Journal of the Royal Historical and Archaeological Association of Ireland* in 1870 but was interrupted by Wilde's work on the 1871 census.[68] During the 1860s he had collected material from Beranger's family connections and his attention was drawn to 'Notes and Anecdotes' – 'a large MS. book of 118 pages, in double columns. It is most beautifully written in a clear, distinct hand, without a blot or erasure, and contains several small illustrative sketches . . .'.

The *Memoir* is an edited version of the 'Notes' amplified by Wilde's inevitable digressions. These include an account of the genealogy of the O'Conor family, some of whom were his father's patients, the faction fights formerly a feature of the 'Pattern day' at Glendalough, and his own boyhood visits on the first of May to the imposing rath at Croghan

when all the great Connaught oxen of the extensive plains around were driven in to be bled, and the peasantry gathered in with pots, turf, bags of meal, and bundles of *scallions* to make 'possets' with the warm blood as it flowed from the shoulders of the beeves, that were soon to find their way from the Baalfes, Taafes, Farrells and Frenches, to swell the coffers of Billy Murphy in Smith-field; where their thick hides formed the buff belts of the soldiery of Europe, and their flesh went to support the navies of Great Britain - 'in the good ould war-times of Boney'.[69]

Wilde admired Beranger's bird paintings and praised his representation of flowers and animals. 'There was one animal he drew to perfection and seemed to delight in it – the good old Irish pig – lengthy, thin, leggy, hog-backed, long-necked, four-eared – his

---

*   See the elegant *Beranger's Views of Ireland*, a Royal Irish Academy publication, with text by Peter Harbison (Dublin 1991).

tail, with a twist and a half in it, and bushy at the end, telegraphing to his knowing, half-shut eye, nearly covered by his long drooping upper lug, and glancing over his flexible, acute snout . . .'.[70] The verbal description is no less masterly than the artist's sketches.

Wilde devotes many pages to his own views on the Irish round towers but disappointingly confines his description of Beranger to 25 lines:

The good old Dutchman was spare in person, of middle height, his natural hair powdered and gathered into a queue; he had a sharp well-cut brow and good bushy eye-brows, divided by the special artistic indentation; a clear, observant, square-ended nose, that sniffed humbug and took in fun; clear, quick, brown eyes; a well-cut, playful, dramatic mouth, eloquent and witty; not a powerful but a chin quite congruent with the face. Well shaven, no shirt to be seen, but his neck surrounded with a voluminous neck cloth, fringed at the ends, a drab, rather quaker-cut coat and vest for household purposes, and when on sketching excursions he had on a long scarlet frock coat and yellow breeches, top boots, a three cocked-hat, and held in his hand a tall staff and a measuring tape. Like Woverman's white horse or Petrie's red woman, he frequently introduced himself in this remarkable but at the time not uncommon costume into his pictures . . .[71]

The *Memoir* was not intended to be a full 'Life'. Like Wilde's other essays in this genre it deals with a selected period of his subject's career, leaving us regretting that the passages of truly splendid prose are not fashioned more fully to form a single narrative entity undisturbed by digressions, and conscious that the author's talents as scholar, scientist and collector clash to the detriment of the biographical art.

He did not live to complete his account of Gabriel Beranger, which was finished by Speranza and published posthumously. He completed his *Report on the 1871 Census* in 1874 but towards the end of the following year his health was failing. 'He faded away gently before our eyes,' Lady Wilde told a friend, 'still trying to work, almost to the last, going down to attend professional duties.'[72] But in March he kept to his bed – 'the last few days he was almost unconscious, quiet and still and at the last passed away like one sleeping', his wife holding his hand and his sons beside him.

He died on 19 April 1876 and was buried in Mount Jerome, a short distance from the grave of his cousin Gideon Ousley. Among those who attended the funeral were Isaac Butt, who

had been leading counsel for Miss Travers, Archibald Jacob, the
son of his enemy Arthur Jacob, who had died two years earlier,
the President of the Royal Irish Academy, accompanied by the
mace-bearer, who carried the mace swathed in crêpe. Many
colleagues stood at the graveside, including Dr Henry Gogarty,
whose son was to use the pen-name Gideon Ousley. Within
days Sir Samuel Ferguson composed an elegy for his friend. His
stanzas, appropriately, were forward-looking:

> Dear Wilde, the deeps close o'er thee; and no more
> Greet we or mingle on the hither shore,
> Where other footsteps now must print the sand,
> And other waiters by the margin stand.[73]

NOTES

1. T. G. Wilson, *Victorian Doctor* (London 1942), p. 296.
2. Henrietta Corkran: cited by Wilson, *op. cit.*, p. 308.
3. Joseph Toynbee (1815–66), aural surgeon to St Mary's Hospital, London,
   and author of *Diseases of the Ear* (1860). His son, Arnold (1852–83), devoted
   his short life to social work and philosophy.
4. William R. Wilde, *Practical Observations on Aural Surgery and the Nature and
   Treatment of Diseases of the Ear* (London 1853), p. 2.
5. Leslie T. Morton, *A Medical Bibliography (Garrison and Morton)* (London
   1970), p. 397.
6. Colm Ó Lochlainn in preface to W. R. Wilde, *The Boyne and the Blackwater*
   (Dublin 1949).
7. Liam de Paor, 'Wilde the Antiquarian', *The Irish Times*, 14 September 1976,
   p. 8.
8. Sir Peter Froggatt, 'Sir William Wilde and the 1851 Census of Ireland',
   Med. Hist. (1965), 9: 306.
9. Terence de Vere White, *The Parents of Oscar Wilde* (London 1976), *passim*.
10. Wilson, *op. cit.*, p. 2.
11. Sir William R. Wilde, *Lough Corrib, Its Shores and Islands* (Dublin 1867),
    p. 156.
12. Sir Charles Cameron, *History of the Royal College of Surgeons of Ireland*
    (Dublin 1886 and 1916), p. 679, p. 836.
13. See Muriel McCarthy's sympathetic account of Travers (*All Graduates &
    Gentlemen* [Dublin 1980]). An unexpected outcome of the libel case was
    that Robert Travers (1807–88) was not promoted when the post of
    Keeper of Marsh's Library fell vacant in 1872. In consequence he gave his
    books to Chetham's Library, Manchester, instead of to Marsh's as intended.
14. Attributed by Wilson (*op. cit.*, p. 273) to Arthur Jacob but he was no longer
    editor. See Davis Coakley, *The Irish School of Medicine* (Dublin 1988), p. 136.
15. William R. Wilde, *Dublin University Magazine* (1841), 18: 305–27; 470–89;
    604–18; 744–63.

16. *Ibid.*, p. 305.
17. *Ibid.*, p. 315.
18. John Flamsteed (1646–1719), the first astronomer royal; Robert Boyle (1627–91), chemist and natural philosopher, enunciated 'Boyle's law'; Robert Hooke (1635–1703), experimental philosopher; Nehemiah Grew (1641–1712), author of *The Anatomy of Plants*.
19. Wilde, *op. cit.*, p. 321.
20. *Ibid.*, p. 323.
21. *Ibid.*, p. 325.
22. *Ibid.*, p. 470.
23. *Ibid.*, p. 475.
24. *Ibid.*, p. 472.
25. *Ibid.*, p. 480.
26. *Ibid.*, p. 483.
27. *Ibid.*, p. 486.
28. *Ibid.*, p. 614.
29. *Ibid.*, p. 764.
30. William R. Wilde, 'Sir Henry Marsh, Bart', *Dublin University Magazine* (1841), 18: 688–92.
31. *Ibid.*, p. 689.
32. *Ibid.*, p. 691.
33. William R. Wilde, 'Robert J. Graves', *Dublin University Magazine* (1842), 19: 260–73.
34. *Ibid.*, p. 262. He published an early account of exophthalmic goitre, commonly called 'Graves's disease'.
35. Sir William R. Wills Wilde, *Biographical Memoir of the Late Robert H. Graves, M.D.* (Dublin 1864). There is no copy of this rare booklet in Dublin. The only copy traced in London (British Library) is incomplete. The first full biography of Graves was written by Selwyn Taylor (London 1989); see also J. B. Lyons, *Brief Lives of Irish Doctors* (Dublin 1978), Nora Robertson, *Crowned Harp* (Dublin 1960), Davis Coakley, *The Irish School of Medicine* (Dublin 1988).
36. *Memoir*, p. 32.
37. *Ibid.*, p. 31.
38. The Standing Committee complained 'that a bargain has been made between two Medical Gentlemen whereby a consideration in money was to be paid on the appointment of a Physician to fill the present Vacancy' and opposed it. The medical board insisted 'that in electing a Gentleman of Doctor Graves' character and qualifications they conceive they have considered the best interests of the Hospital'. *Hospital Minutes*, Meath Hospital.
39. Wilde, *Dublin University Magazine* (1842), 42: 273.
40. Andrew K. Young in Appendix to *Medical History of the Meath Hospital* by Lambert H. Ormsby (Dublin 1892), pp. 34–45.
41. Cameron, *op. cit.*, p. 590.
42. William R. Wilde, 'Sir Robert Kane, M.D.', *Dublin University Magazine* (1849), 33: 626–37.

43. *Ibid.*, p. 628.
44. Minutes of the King and Queen's College of Physicians, 19 September 1833, p. 198.
45. *Ibid.*, 26 October 1840, p. 400. Kane was elected fellow in 1841.
46. Wilde, *op. cit.*, p. 634.
47. *Ibid.*, p. 637.
48. [William R. Wilde], 'Bartholomew Mosse, M.D.', *Dublin Quarterly Journal of Medical Science* (1846), 2: 565–96.
49. *Ibid.*, p. 571.
50. *Ibid.*, p. 572.
51. *Ibid.*, p. 587.
52. *Ibid.*, p. 588.
53. *Ibid.*, p. 591. His widow's petition resulted in a grant of £1000. Jane Mosse, by whom he had two children, was a daughter of Archdeacon Whittingham. She was his second wife. Elizabeth Mary Mallory, his first wife, died childless within a short time of their marriage.
54. [William R. Wilde], 'John Oliver Curran, M.B.', *Dublin Quarterly Journal of Medical Science* (1847), 4: 500–12.
55. *Ibid.*, p. 500.
56. *Ibid.*, p. 511.
57. [William R. Wilde], 'Sylvester O'Halloran, M.R.I.A.', *Dublin Quarterly Journal of Medical Science* (1848), 6: 223–32.
58. W. J. Mc Cormack, 'Sylvester O'Halloran and Maria Edgeworth's *Absentee*', *Long Room* (1974), No. 9: 41.
59. William R. Wilde, 'Some Particulars respecting Swift and Stella', *Dublin Quarterly Journal of Medical Science* (1847), 3: 334–438 and 4: 1–33.
60. See T. G. Wilson, 'Swift's Deafness and Last Illness', *Irish Journal of Medical Science* (1939), 241–56 and Sir Walter Russell Brain, *ibid.* (1952), 337–45. The retrospective diagnosis of Ménière's disease was suggested by J. C. Bucknill in the neurological journal *Brain* in January 1882 but Dr J. Wickham Legg claimed priority for his article in *The Academy* (1881), 19: 475.
61. William R. Wilde, *The Closing Years of Dean Swift's Life*, 2nd ed. (Dublin 1849), p. 53.
62. *Ibid.*, p. 121.
63. *Ibid.*, p. 76.
64. Wilson, *Victorian Doctor*, pp. 156–60.
65. William R. Wilde, 'Some Account of Richard Steevens, M.D., and his Hospital', *Medical Times and Gazette*, 6 December 1856, 565–6.
66. *Ibid.*, 566.
67. *Ibid.*, 566.
68. 'Memoir of Gabriel Beranger, and his labours in the cause of Irish art, literature and antiquities, from 1760 to 1780. With an illustration of the Round Tower of St Michael le Pole, Dublin', *Journal of Royal Historical and Architectural Association of Ireland*, series 4, 1870, 1: 33–64, 121–52, 236–60; 1873, 2: 445–85; 1876, 4: 111–56.

69. *Memoir of Gabriel Beranger* (Dublin 1880), p. 49.
70. *Ibid*., p. 29.
71. *Ibid*., p. 28.
72. Larcom correspondence, NLI, cited by T. de V. White, *op. cit.*, p. 228.
73. 'Dear Wilde. An Elegy, 1876', *Poems by Sir Samuel Ferguson* (Dublin 1880), pp. 164–6. During Wilde's editorship the *Dublin Quarterly Journal of Medical Science* published biographical articles on John Houston and Bryan Higgins by R. G. Butcher and W. K. Sullivan respectively; also an article on James Houghton MD (obituary), possibly by the editor. The National Union Catalogue lists a *Life and Times of George Robert Fitzgerald, commonly called Fighting Fitzgerald* under Wilde's authorship (Dublin 1852). The evidence for the attribution is unclear, other than the fact that the copy is bound with Wilde's *Irish Popular Superstitions*, which would explain the error.

5

'What did I die of?' – The Last Illness of Charles Stewart Parnell*

CHARLES Stewart Parnell's death at forty-five on 6 October 1891 was sudden and unexpected. A few weeks previously, the *Connaught Telegraph* had intimated with inconceivable malice that he should follow the example of Castlereagh, who cut his throat. There were rumours in London in October that he had, indeed, committed suicide. Others believed that he was still alive. As late as 1896, Mrs Delia Parnell held that her son had either been assassinated by British agents or was still living; John Dillon thought he saw and heard him in Munich at a performance of *Götterdämmerung*; St John Ervine[1] was told in Belfast during the Boer War that General de Wet was really the disguised Irish statesman.

Despite these rumours Parnell's biographers have, in the main, avoided the task of reviewing his last illness in terms of modern pathology with the hope of arriving at a more acceptable diagnosis than that offered by Jowers, the doctor in attendance. From the viewpoint of biography it may not matter greatly what a man dies from; the general circumstances of the death and who stands by the bedside are far more relevant. And yet the theatrical appropriateness of Parnell's death in the eye of the storm demands an explanation.

When researching his magisterial biography, the late F.S.L. Lyons[2] did consider the matter. The former provost of Trinity College sought the advice of a colleague in the Medical School who offered a diagnosis of lobar pneumonia, then a common and lethal disease, and ascribed the pain in 'the damaged left arm' to

* A Thomas Davis Lecture broadcast from Radio Éireann on 13 January 1985.

rheumatism. This is certainly a possible explanation but does not give sufficient weight to what is actually the presenting symptom and overlooks the family history.

'Whoever heard', Parnell's mother asked with consuming sarcasm, 'of rheumatism passing from a man's left arm and killing him in a single night?'

Her scepticism would be out of place today: the pain of coronary heart disease can be confined to one or other arm yet presage coronary thrombosis and cardiac arrest which may slay in an instant.

FAMILY HISTORY

Medical diagnosis is facilitated nowadays by laboratory aids inapplicable to Parnell's case but still depends largely on an analysis of the 'presenting complaint' considered against the background of the patient's health record and that of his family. The Parnells of Avondale, an Anglo-Irish family, had roots in Cheshire and Queen's County. The first of the line for whom relevant medical data are available is Sir John Parnell, the second baronet. Sir Jonah Barrington described him as 'a large, casual, untidy kind of man'. He was given to the pleasures of the table and died suddenly 'at the height of his exaltation' aged fifty-seven. His third son, William, who inherited Avondale, was MP for Wicklow; while in Dublin on business in January 1821 'he caught the chill which led to his death'. He was then only forty-four years of age and left two children, Catherine and John Henry.

By his marriage to a beautiful American girl, Delia Tudor Stewart, John Henry Parnell had eleven children. The eldest, William Tudor, died 'through bad vaccination' at a tender age; Hayes, the second son, succumbed to tuberculosis in early adolescence. John Howard enjoyed a long life and died in 1923; as a youngster he stammered and through mimicry his younger brother, Charles Stewart, the subject of this article, almost acquired a speech defect. Henry, the youngest son, was too nervous to pass his law examinations at Cambridge and spent much of his adult life travelling to improve his health.

Delia, the eldest daughter, a notable dark beauty, married for money and lived to regret it, making at least one attempt at suicide. Emily's romance with a wild young neighbour, Arthur Dickinson, displeased her father, who forbade it. Sophia, a blonde beauty, was to elope with the family solicitor at sixteen; she died at thirty-two having nursed her children through scarlet fever. Fanny, the poet of the family, experienced a breakdown in health in the 1870s; she died suddenly at Bordenstown, New Jersey in 1882. Anna was drowned in 1911 having gone swimming against advice on a stormy day at Ilfracombe. Theodosia, the youngest child, married an English naval officer and lived a happy and uneventful life.

John Henry Parnell, the father of the family, was a conventional squire with a liking for outdoor sport, in particular cricket. Towards the end of June 1859, against the advice of Sir Henry Marsh, a leading physician, he insisted on keeping an engagement to play for Leinster Cricket Club against Phoenix although suffering from what was euphemistically termed 'rheumatism of the stomach'. During his visit to Dublin he also called on his solicitor to disinherit Emily, angered by news from London that she was on the point of eloping with Dickinson.

The combination of physical exertion and emotional strain was too much for the ailing man, who was taken acutely ill in the Shelbourne Hotel after the cricket match and died there on 3 July. As he was then only forty-eight years old the most likely diagnosis is myocardial infarction, a disorder then unknown to medical practitioners. It is possible that his father and grandfather were also victims of the disease, which was recognized with increasing frequency after the publication of James B. Herrick's article 'Clinical features of sudden obstruction of the coronary arteries' in the *Journal of the American Medical Association* in 1912.

HEALTH RECORD

Born in Avondale on 27 June 1846, Charles Stewart Parnell grew up in circumstances conducive to good health but exposed like all his contemporaries to the constant threat of infectious illness. At an early age he contracted typhoid fever in school at Yeovil. This appears to have been followed by emotional or nervous instability, for his parents took him to London to be seen by Dr Forbes Winslow, a Cavendish Square alienist, author of *Health and Body and Mind*. Later he was laid up with scarlet fever.

John Howard Parnell[3] described his brother as 'a wiry little boy . . . very small for his age' and nicknamed Tom Thumb. He enjoyed outdoor games, shooting and fishing but was highly strung and when watching cricket his fingers twitched anxiously. In the 1860s he was an enthusiastic supporter of the local hunt but when a doctor told him, erroneously, that he had a weak heart he gave up hunting. When in America in 1871 he was lucky to escape serious injury when his train jumped the rails. He sustained a hand injury in the quarry at Avondale and Sir Alfred Robbins[4] recalled that in 1889 he appeared on a public platform with his left arm in a sling, having burned it in the course of a chemistry experiment. At Castlecomer a bag of lime thrown by a political enemy burst in his face and Dr J. Byrne Hackett found him sitting in the carriage in great pain.

Like many young men he drank heavily. He was sent down from Cambridge after involvement in a drunken brawl and in September 1869 he and his alcoholic brother-in-law, Captain Arthur Dickinson, were charged with disorderly conduct at the Glendalough Hotel. This phase was temporary. R.F. Foster[5] cites a newspaper reporter's interview at Avondale in 1880: 'Mr Parnell is very abstemious, drinking little but water and tea. He smokes a great deal and is never in want of a good "weed" which he proffers very liberally to his friends . . .'. Mr Foster adds that Parnell reduced his smoking under Mrs O'Shea's influence but clearly did not eschew it completely; St John Ervine describes how Parnell spent some hours after the split with Justin McCarthy, who recalled: 'He was as friendly and as familiar as if nothing whatever had occurred to divide us, and we smoked at intervals of work and drank whiskey and soda . . .'.[6] He appears to have enjoyed his meals, though neither a sybarite nor an ascetic, and by doctor's orders drank still Moselle with dinner.

A description of Parnell in his maturity is given by Katharine O'Shea:

When I first met Mr Parnell in 1880 he was unusually tall and very thin. His features were delicate with that pallid pearly tint of skin that was always pecu-liarly his. The shadows under his deep sombre eyes made them appear larger than they were, and the eyes themselves were the most striking features of his cold, handsome face.[7]

John Howard Parnell also mentioned his brother's gauntness – 'except during a period from about 1885 to 1890, when he became rather stout' – which combined with his striking pallor to convey an impression of frailty. This was belied by a resilience which enabled him to endure long hours and to travel in the bitterest weather. Standish O'Grady[8] remembered encountering him on an outside car on a dreadfully cold day in 1891. 'Parnell was muffled in the most copious manner, quite a hill of rugs, cloaks and shawls.'

Temperamentally he was highly-strung, superstitious, aggressive and prone to nightmares and sleepwalking. He was not a natural orator and in his early days as a public speaker dug his nails into his palms when facing the audience. While in Kilmainham Jail he was treated by his colleague, Dr Joseph Kenny, Nationalist MP for Cork, for a series of minor ailments. The reliability of the health record for this period is vitiated by the need, as he explained to Mrs O'Shea, 'to invent little maladies for myself from day to day in order to give Dr Kenny an excuse for keeping me in the infirmary, but I have never felt better in my life'.[9]

On the eve of a meeting of the National League in October 1882 he had an acute attack of 'dysenterical diarrhoea'. Four years later when more seriously ill he consulted a leading London surgeon, Sir Henry Thompson. It is improbable that Parnell had Bright's disease, a serious kidney disease mentioned by some biographers. This diagnosis may be based on the fact that Sir Henry was a pioneer urologist, but in her book Mrs O'Shea stated unequivocally that her lover had a nervous breakdown brought on by overwork.[10] One point of physical importance emerges from the visit to Sir Henry Thompson: the surgeon's observation that Parnell's circulation was bad.

Like many public figures he was the victim of sensation-mongers. The newspapers once carried the news of his 'assassination'; on an another occasion he was reported to be in an insane asylum in Spain. During the debate on the first Home Rule bill the rumour of his death spread from Dublin. 'What did I die of?' Parnell asked on hearing of the latest falsehood.

PRESENTING COMPLAINT

The solace afforded by Parnell's marriage to Mrs Katharine O'Shea on 25 June 1891 cannot have fully mitigated for him the effect of the political ordeals. By September he seemed exhausted but his wife could not prevail upon him to visit Sir Henry Thompson when passing through London. Towards the end of the month Parnell wrote to Dr Kenny from his Dublin headquarters, Morrison's Hotel, asking him to call. He was suffering from what R. Barry O'Brien[11] referred to as 'acute rheumatism and general debility' and carried his left arm in a sling. Dr Kenny advised him not to attend a meeting in Creggs but Parnell insisted on doing so.

On his return to Dublin, Parnell stayed with Dr Kenny for a few days. 'He looked ill and fatigued, ate little and suffered from acute rheumatic pains in the hand and arm.' Against the doctor's advice he left for England on Wednesday, 30 September. He took a Turkish bath in London and went on to Brighton, fated to die shortly before midnight on 6 October, without realizing that he was mortally ill.

On his arrival at 9 Walsingham Terrace on Thursday, 1 October, he appeared so weak that he was helped into the house by his wife. He ate a fairly good dinner and rested before a blazing fire. Eventually, using a stick, he went up to bed; his wife rubbed him with firwood oil and packed the left arm with wool. Next morning he stayed in bed but enjoyed his breakfast, smoked a cigar and made notes for a speech. He refused to send for Sir Henry Thompson on the grounds of expense but wrote to him, expecting an early reply. He wrote, too, to his solicitor about a mortgage and to Dr Kenny, secretary of a committee set up to provide a home for James Stephens, the elderly Fenian.[12]

On Sunday he was depressed and unwell. His wife insisted on calling a local practitioner, being uneasy about the pain. When Parnell had spoken to Dr Jowers he felt better but slept badly that night and was feverish. He still refused to summon the Wimpole Street specialist and on Monday afternoon received a letter from London. 'You see, sweetheart, I was right,' he said to Mrs Parnell when she read Sir Henry's letter. 'Thompson says just what Jowers does; there's no need to have him down.' He decided it was unnecessary to call Dr Willoughby Furner, whom Sir Henry recommended, having confidence in Jowers.

He was in great pain on Monday and experienced, too, what his wife described as 'a sudden horror that he was being held down by some strong unseen power'. He attempted to get out of bed but was too weak to stand. A sleepless night followed and on Tuesday he was flushed and feverish but content to accept the doctor's explanation that improvement could not be expected for some days. Dr Jowers came again later in the day and promised to call early next morning.

The last moments of her husband's life have been described by Mrs Parnell:

Late in the evening he suddenly opened his eyes and said: 'Kiss me, sweet Wifie, and I will try to sleep a little.' I lay down by his side and kissed the burning lips he pressed to mine for the last time. The fire of them, fierce beyond any I had ever felt, even in his most loving moods, startled me, and as I slipped my hand from under his head he gave a little sigh and became unconscious. The doctor came at once, but no remedies prevailed against this sudden failure of the heart's action, and my husband died without regaining consciousness.[13]

The body of their dead leader was seen by Dr J. G. Fitzgerald, Henry Harrison and others but Mrs Emily Dickinson, the bereaved sister, was not permitted to view the remains on account of the early onset of signs of post-mortem decay.

DIFFERENTIAL DIAGNOSIS

Sir Henry Thompson's letters of sympathy to the widow expressed shock and distress at the unexpected turn of events together with the consolation that nothing had been left undone. 'I doubt', he wrote, 'whether anything would have saved him when passing through London. A blow had been struck – not so heavy – apparently a light one; but his worn-out constitution . . . had no power to resist . . . Dr Jowers is an experienced and most capable man, and I think you may rest assured that he could scarcely have been in safer hands.'[14]

Sir Henry's generalities bring no enlightenment as to the nature of the pathology and Dr Jowers obviously was equally at sea but issued a certificate that death was caused by 'rheumatic fever 5 days, hyperpyrexia, failure of the heart's action'. James B. Herrick's vital paper was still unpublished.

It has, incidentally, been stated that Parnell was attended by Dr Benjamin (*sic*) Jowers, junior, but the Medical Directory shows that Dr Jowers and his father were named Lancelot Emilius and Frederic William respectively. The former was then only three years qualified whereas Sir Henry Thompson referred to an experienced man and the death certificate was signed by F. W. Jowers FRCS. This suggests that when young Dr Jowers realized how ill the notability under his care really was he prudently called his father.

THE DIAGNOSIS

The diagnosis of pneumonia offered in the late F.S.L. Lyons's biography seems to me unlikely other than as a terminal complication. Lobar pneumonia has a characteristic clinical picture and was then a commonplace which would have been readily recognized by Dr Jowers. According to Sir William Osler a patient with lobar pneumonia presented a picture 'more distinctive than that presented by any other acute disease'.[15]

The evidence of Bright's disease referred to by Sir Alfred Robbins is almost equally unconvincing. Lung cancer with involvement of the brachial plexus or a prolapsed cervical intervertebral disc are conditions to be included in the differential diagnosis; neither would be expected to terminate in cardiac arrest so characteristic of myocardial infarction, which emerges as the probable diagnosis.

There remains to be fitted into the clinical mosaic, hyperpyrexia, the excessively high fever which is a feature of heatstroke and a occasional occurrence in fulminating infections and brainstem haemorrhage. Heatstroke is not, of course, a reality to be considered in an English autumn. It is conceivable that Parnell had a terminal septicaemia but a brain lesion would seem a more likely explanation. The crux of the matter, however, is its lack of credibility. The doctors, floundering in an adverse situation, left no reliable data.[16] Has this clinical statement any more authority than the rumour that William Parnell died following a chill or that John Henry Parnell played cricket when running a temperature? The alleged need for hurried coffining in a lead-lined casket, too, savours more of a mystery story than a reality.

According to Henry Harrison, who was present, Parnell's body was not placed in the coffin until Friday night. 'The final closing was deferred until the morrow . . . the heavy leaden casket was sealed up and, in its turn, shut in within a massive oaken coffin of unusual design.'[17]

PROGNOSIS

Biographers are not afforded the freedom enjoyed by novelists but they are not expected to adopt the exactitudes of legal terminology or to accept the restraints of clinical science. This may explain why Parnell's biographers, presumably to suit the direction of their narratives, have invariably invested their descriptions of the care-worn parliamentarian with a taint of moribundity. Such rehearsals of doom are missing from *The Last Five Years* by Sir Alfred Robbins, in which Parnell is portrayed as capable of a degree of activity hardly to be expected if he were in the last stages of a debilitating illness:

Having on the night of his arrival addressed a wildly enthusiastic meeting in the Rotunda, he rose early the next morning, and, before starting for Cork, launched personally an attack on the offices of United Ireland, which had gone over to his opponents. Finding them barred against him he followed the example of the Lion Heart at the gates of Front de Boeuf's castle, and with a crowbar battered his way through the front door; helped to throw out the members of the staff; and pale, dishevelled, covered with dust, presented himself at an upstairs window, and ringingly declared, 'I rely on Dublin. Dublin is true.'[18]

On a later page, Robbins provides another picture of a man taxed to the limits of endurance but not beyond the remedial powers of *vis medicatrix naturae*:

He was so tireless in his energy as to alarm his friends, who warned him of the certain result; but he hated the suggestion of unfitness to stand the continuous strain. More than once, when he would pass through the Lobby that spring and summer, looking harassed and weary and unlike his old self, he assured me he was enjoying the fight. Justin McCarthy, with whom he had resumed friendly personal relations, exclaimed to him one evening, 'Parnell, are you not overdoing this? No constitution can stand the work you are going through.' 'I like it,' he replied. 'It is doing me a lot of good' – the last words his old friend heard him speak. 'I am doing the work of ten men', he told another intimate: 'but it does me good.'[19]

Paul Bew, the latest biographer, has stated that when Parnell returned to Brighton 'he was clearly on his last legs'.[20] Events

have appeared to justify the colloquialism, which is acceptable
only as a retrospective judgment – without some knowledge of
the attendant pathology that prognostic statement, applied to a
man of forty-five, is unwarranted. What if Dr Kenny's advice
had been followed? Might not Parnell, to use another non-
clinical phrase, have got his second wind? If my submission is
correct and the left arm pain was evidence of 'coronary insuf-
ficiency', insistence on rest, avoidance of the testing meeting at
Creggs and a prolonged convalescence might have at least postponed the dire consequences that ensued. But Charles Stewart
Parnell, no less stubborn than his cricketing father and equally
heedless of medical advice, insisted on having his own way, with
the same sad result.

NOTES

1. St John Ervine, *Parnell* (London 1928), p. 293.
2. F.S.L. Lyons, *Charles Stewart Parnell* (London 1977), *passim*.
3. John Howard Parnell, *Charles Stewart Parnell: A Memoir* (London 1916), *passim*.
4. Sir Alfred Robbins, *Parnell: The Last Five Years* (London 1926), p. 106.
5. R.F. Foster, *Charles Stewart Parnell – The Man and his Family* (Hassocks 1976), p. 186.
6. Ervine, *op. cit.*, p. 311.
7. K. O'Shea, *Charles Stewart Parnell: His Love Story and Political Life*, vol. 2 (London 1914), p. 238.
8. Standish O'Grady, *The Story of Ireland* (London 1894), p. 203.
9. Lyons, *op. cit.*, p. 185.
10. O'Shea, *op. cit.*, p. 46.
11. R. B. O'Brien, *The Life of Charles Stewart Parnell*, vol. 2 (London 1898), p. 349.
12. M. Leamy, *Parnell's Faithful Few* (New York 1936), p. 102.
13. O'Shea, *op. cit.*, p. 275.
14. *Ibid.*, p. 273.
15. Sir William Osler, *The Principles and Practice of Medicine* (London 1909), p. 172.
16. One suspects that 'hyperpyrexia', i.e. a temperature of 106° F or higher, was a conjectural figment of Dr Jowers's imagination in response to the distraught widow's reference to 'the burning lips . . . ' rather than an actual diagnosis based on a thermometer reading. Had Dr Jowers recorded a temperature of that level during the illness he would have been bound to mention it to Mrs Parnell, who would surely have referred to it in her book.

17. H. Harrison, *Parnell Vindicated* (London 1931), p. 97.
18. Robbins, *op. cit.*, p. 180.
19. *Ibid.*, p. 189.
20. Paul Bew, *C.S. Parnell* (Dublin 1980), p. 134.

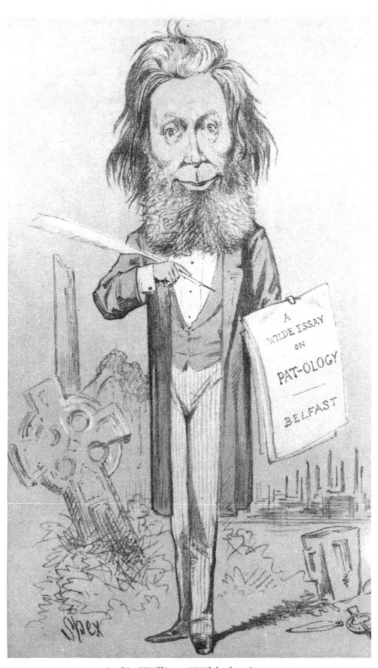

4. Sir William Wilde by Spex

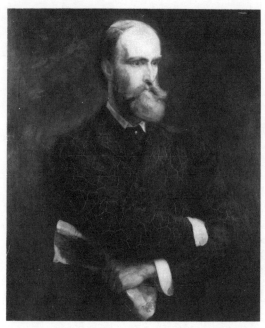

5. Charles Stewart Parnell by Sydney Hall (Courtesy of the National Gallery of Ireland)

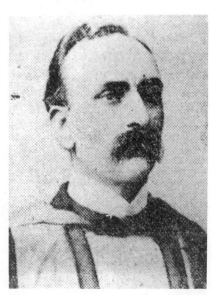

6. Dr John Knott (From the *Freeman's Journal*)

6

A Forgotten Scholar: John
Freeman Knott, 1853–1921*

THE term 'para-medical writers' could be applied to authors who,
while following careers in medicine, have written extensively on
historical and literary aspects of their profession. Their essays are
generally destined for medical journals, thus existing in a limbo
removed from the main body of letters, though a modicum of
general recognition may be attained by larger reference works.
Prominent Irish exponents of the genre (living authors excluded)
were James Henry, Sir William Wilde, Sir Charles Cameron,
T.P.C. Kirkpatrick, William Doolin, J.D.H. Widdess and Patrick
Logan.[1] A largely forgotten name should be added to the list, that
of Dr John Knott.

After his death in 1921, Knott was accorded laudatory obituaries[2]
but he is unknown to recent generations with the exception of
those curious readers who recall an arresting vignette contributed
by Widdess in a passage which describes how the insurgents
advanced on the College of Surgeons on Easter Monday, 1916:

At the same time Dr John Knott, an elderly, erudite and eccentric Fellow of
the College, whose daughter Eleanor[3] became a noted Celtic scholar, set out
for the College. Ignoring the sounds of battle, unscathed by flying bullets, he
arrived at the front door of his College, in the Library of which he was
accustomed to spend his day in study, composing learned communications on
subjects ranging from female circumcision to spontaneous combustion. The
bedel, who had observed from a window his approach through York Street,
answered the doctor's knock. Frank Robbins and his party seized the opportunity. The door was opened slightly to tell Dr Knott that the College had
been closed by order of the Registrar. As the bedel related, before he could
shut the door the Countess Markievicz with 'two other rebels presented themselves at the Hall door, one of the rebels firing at close range a rifle' at him.[4]

* Published in *Long Room*, No. 34 (1989), 31–46.

We do not learn how Knott reacted to the situation but
'elderly' is a relative term – he was then in his sixty-third year
and in possession of all his wits. A contemporary, a librarian who
shared Knott's tastes, described him as 'courteous and affable . . .
He was the proud possessor of a large and valuable collection of
unique books; and it was a rare treat to hear him discourse on
the history of early printing or describe some anecdote in connexion with a rare volume which he would sometimes take from
his library.'[5]

I

John Freeman Knott was the only son of William Knott, a
County Roscommon farmer and bailiff to the local landlord.[6] He
was born at Kingsland, near Frenchpark, on 5 June 1853, and
educated at the local National School. He had private lessons in
Latin and Greek from Dean Burke of Boyle and also learned,
then or later, how to read French, German, Italian and Spanish.
He married at twenty; his bride was Elizabeth Shera of Boyle.

Information about the formative years is lacking but a journal
or diary which John Knott kept through 1874 and his letters to
his wife from Dublin (she is 'E' in the journal and 'Bessie' in the
letters) show that the bookish youth was already a practical
farmer.

When the journal opens in 1874, William Knott is seventy-six
and has been operated on by Sir William Wilde for cataracts.
John Knott appears to be in charge of the 45-acre family farm at
Kingsland and Tonroe, and is bailiff to the King Harmans with
responsibility for collection of rents and evictions. The first entry
on 6 January refers to a visit on New Year's Day to the Rent
Office in Boyle where tenants were expected: 'The Rents were
smartly raised as they found out then.' Captain King-Harman
bade young Knott a civil good morning but his son ignored him.
Subsequent entries record tasks that are a farmer's common lot
but this is an uncommon farmer. 'Read during the 2 last evenings
about i page of Dante and other little things & an epigram of
Martial.'

Jan 15. Day wet, so that I had no man. Accordingly after breakfast I started out
rent-warning . . . Got a good wetting of course. After dinner and regulating

things about home I took a trip to Tonroe (in the dusk). Had a grand evening of it, the old pair took tea with us and E played and sang a good deal. I read, Goethe, Faust 1½ pages, Homer, Iliad, Book 2, 22 first lines, Blaines, Vet. Pref. Intr and Sect 1–3. Also pieces of poetry.

Jan 16. A mild soft morning, showers of snow in the evening. Sh & P.C. worked here all day and I attended the latter, went nowhere. Read Goethe, Faust, 2 pages (even). Homer, Iliad, II, 23–42. Pieces of English poetry. Tried to commit Poe's 'Raven' to memory.

Through the pages of the journal we accompany John Knott to market along frosty roads with a firkin of butter or to the forge to get hind shoes for Robin, the horse. We are made privy to his worries – 'was gloomy all day fretting about my income as I feared E's improvidence' (23 January) – and join the couple in a tender domestic moment when he is unwell. 'Feb. 18. Ash Wednesday. E bathed my back and thighs last night in "Salt & water" which gave me intense pleasure during the operation and great relief afterwards.' We go with him to the fair at Boyle or with the lengthening days make the longer journey to Roscommon.

Apr. 25. Started for Roscommon at about 3½ a.m. Brought Sh with me. Was there a few minutes before 10. After a short time, I bought 4 ewe lambs from Scally the jobber @ 17/6 each and left town without any delay . . . Arrived at home about 7½ p.m. Gave Sh a glass of whiskey to climb up a tree . . . for cones as I knew E liked them. Put the lambs into the barn for the night, and gave them a little milk.

Apr. 26. Sabbath. Was up early to suckle the lambs. Succeeded admirably with all but one . . . The day was lovely and the night if possible still more so. *Heard the corncrake.*

Apr. 27. Had no workman. Day fine as usual. Spent the greater part of the day at my hot bed. Searched for the stalks which were not up, put bone meal on six ridges . . . Took evening walk with E. and Wally which I enjoyed very much.

Apr. 29. Another lovely day, Mary found Strawberry calved, a beautiful heifer. I was in high delight but alas for worldly joys my eckstasies were soon afterwards calmed down on the intelligence that the bullock which came from Boyle was dead.

John and Elizabeth Knott appear to have been a little at odds with the old folk who may have nursed grievances that follow the surrender of power and the arrival of a new wife.

Got a good deal of annoyance at night. I overheard the old fellow muttering to himself . . . I overheard him asserting his exclusive claim to the place, land stock and all, stigmatising the blackguard conduct etc. I was sickened with rage and vexation. I had to lie on the bed. When mother who had been out came in I spoke to her in savage style about the matter, which took him down completely.

The elders retired to their own quarters. They were coaxed out with difficulty some days later to declare an uneasy truce. His bickering parents need not have worried him unduly, however, for by now he appears confirmed in his decision to study medicine – on 15 May he is reading Carpenter's *Textbook of Physiology*. This decision, as we shall see, was not made lightly nor does it appear to have lessened in the slightest his enthusiasm for current tasks.

June 5. Got a pleasant surprise from dear E in the morn. She rose in the morning in her night dress 2 or 3 times and at last succeeded in finding under the bed 'Purdon's Practical Farmer' a birthday gift for me. She was well hugged in return, but alas for human pleasures, a few minutes after A. Mulrooney came to the door with the cattle which he had found in his oats.

A brief visit to Howard Hall near Clifden necessitated a round-about journey through Galway via Mullingar, where he missed his connection and waited for the evening train. 'Saw a drunken trull at the station and (shame to say) I felt the old serpent move me of course I overcame the temptation, but it should not have been so.'

On 10 June he ordered Gray's *Anatomy* which he read on summer evenings having drawn turf from the bog, planted cabbage, saved the hay and sent cows to the bull. 'Read Virgil 102–409 Gray (Introduction) general anat and 1st sentence on the Blood' (19 June). 'Read Gray – end of general anat. Virgil Aeneid V 1–102' (5 July).

The rising winds threatened the wheat crop.

Sept. 2. Day began to be very rough about 12 oc. They alarmed me saying that the oats would all be shed. I roamed about in a kind of despair and at last got 2 men who reaped well till evening . . . Was very happy when the work was going well but was again annoyed when they left some undone in the evening (for they dallied). Read Lucian D 23 (finished) D 24, over a page.

During a holiday in Sligo he visited the Town Hall – 'looking over the Directory for the addresses of the Registrar of the principal medical colleges' – but the approaching adventure caused much heart-searching.

Sept. 24. Stayed at home. Day fine. Strolled to Tonroe, spent a good part of the day with the men . . . Came home and raked rushes. Spent a fretful unhappy day. The prospect of going in for the 'Doctoring' trade is now poisoning everything for me. God direct me and strengthen me. Amen. Read Lucian, Timin about 2pp – Macaulay, Walpole about 2 pp (after going to bed).

He dosed a sick calf on 24 October and then set off for Dublin to see the Registrar of the Royal College of Surgeons in Ireland.

He seemed to take a great interest in my case, advised me what to do, introduced me to Dr W.J. Stoker,[7] who took me to his home . . . It was on the whole a very successful day for me. [He returned on 27 October.] Had to walk home from Boyle, but was taken up on the road by my friend P. Kennedy. Met with a hearty welcome from the old people both (which is rare) and my dear E. Found everything very well. The sick calf was as I had left her.

He took his wife to Boyle on Hallowe'en. They met her parents, cracked nuts and chatted about 'the prospects of a medical profession upon which mother looks much distrustfully and father with high ambition'. The next few weeks would have seemed interminable to young Knott.

Nov. 21. The dreaded day has at length arrived. It was very wet. After preparing everything I bid the old pair goodbye, told them I was going from home but did not say whither. Ma in the room combing her hair (she began to snivel at the announcement) Dad in the kitchen corner asked me 'whereto'. I replied that I would tell him when I came back and tore away. P Harrington came with me to bring home the cart . . . Was very miserable leaving Boyle station. Began to cheer up brightly when about halfway. Got sleepy, chilly and sad again towards the end . . . Such is life and I suppose at least such is mine. Alternate joy and sorrow sunshine and shade. Lord be with me and strengthen me for the great conflict.

That afternoon Bessie Knott, who planned to run the place with local labour in her husband's absence, wrote to say how things stood at Kingsland:

Father and Mother break down now and again but are not cross at me though they leave a good deal of the blame on my Father, but particularly on my Mother, also myself.

The weather was so damp the Murrays went home but Pat returned again and is now churning. I take those few moments to let you know how we are getting on before I am called to the butter. The cart has not returned yet but if it comes before the Post Man comes I will let you know.

Now keep up your spirits, trust in God and be careful when attending Hospital, and all will be right . . .

She was kind to the old pair and read out parts of his letters to her father-in-law – 'he does be so anxious to hear from you'. She also described the neighbourhood's reaction to her husband's disappearance:

Dr Irwin,[8] A. Irwin's son, asked Mrs Freeman about your 'Elopement' and she said you intended to be a Dr but she expected you would not be long learning as you had read several Drs Books. He said if such was the case you would not be long until you would be home again with us. Dear me how you have made people talk.

'I get on better than I ever hoped,' Knott assured her, 'for my mind is always occupied.' Their correspondence allows us to follow Knott's progress at the College of Surgeons, seeing him gain confidence as his bright mind placed him at the head of his class. He had digs at 12 Upper Camden Street and walked daily to the Richmond Hospital: 'So you see I am not likely to want for exercise. I must walk backwards and forwards with all speed I can assume for the clinical course begins at 9 O'C and the College lectures at 12.'

The annual introductory lecture delivered by Professor Little[9] impressed young Knott, who was disgusted by the students' rowdy behaviour as they greeted the arrival of College dignitaries. He bought a half-set of bones for £1 and a case of dissecting instruments for nine shillings and Stoker generously gave him a sovereign to replenish his depleted resources. The most notable extra-curricular activities were the services at St Patrick's Cathedral, the visit to Dublin of Moody and Sankey, and Barry Sullivan's *Othello* at the Theatre Royal.

His teachers at the Richmond Hospital included Mr (later Sir) William Stokes[10] – 'son of *the* Stokes of Merrion Square . . . Stokes Jnr is evidently an excellent surgeon as his cases (of amputation, fractures, abscesses, etc.) are almost all progressing favourably. He is also very gentle and tender.' Professor (later Sir Charles) Cameron left a less favourable impression – 'a dull most unintellectual chap, bustling about from one side of the laboratory to another and confusing the various operations of the different students'.[11]

He spent many hours in the dissecting-room and excelled in anatomy. He stayed on in the city to dissect until close to Christmas, increasingly aware of the long separation from Bessie.

'We will have a hot race into one another's arms, I hope, in a few days. They will not be long slipping round.'

When Knott sat for the Mapother Prize in March 1875, the professor said that he had never before encountered such perfect answers.[12] The victorious student called to Mapother's house in Merrion Square to collect the prize and sent it to Kingsland. 'Here is my medal to dearest Bessie. I hope it will give you some pleasure to see it.'

Springtime was unsettling for a displaced countryman but he enjoyed after-dinner walks in St Stephen's Green: 'lovely now with the beautiful hawthorns white and crimson interspersed in full bloom and odour'. He was not allowed to forget the major part Bessie played in the enterprise. If he tended to do so, apologies were required as shown by the following example of his patronizing peacemaking: 'So there's a good child don't be vexed. There are kisses, one, two, three . . . There's a darling – Now don't be grieving or vexed. You are my own pet: there's another kiss.'

The academic session 1875–6 saw Knott appointed to the rank of pro-dissector. It amused him to reflect that on his arrival in the College he had looked up to the pro-dissectors as he might have done to the surgeons-in-ordinary to the Queen. He moved to 21 Charlemont Place, where his rooms were 'sumptuous'. He attended a course in the practice of midwifery at the Coombe Hospital – this entailed 'the additional delights of sitting up 2 nights per week at the Coombe'.

Sir William Wilde, a native of County Roscommon, died on 19 April 1876. 'I did not see Sir W. Wilde's funeral,' he told Bessie, 'but I have heard it was a large one. He was buried in Mount Jerome.'

Knott attended the Pathological Society assiduously and while still a student was awarded its gold medal for a monograph which Fannin published in 1878, *An Essay on the Pathology of the Oesophagus*.

II

Having taken the conjoint diploma of the Irish Colleges of Physicians and Surgeons in May 1877, Knott visited leading Euro-

pean medical centres and held a resident post at the Richmond
Hospital. He registered his qualifications on 12 October 1878
and looked about for a suitable residence. As if providentially, 34
York Street close to the College of Surgeons was vacant. He
settled there, waited for patients and established himself as a
medical crammer.

The Roscommon lands were set at conacre and, writing about
rent, his friend and former neighbour Pat Murray expressed the
hope 'that Mrs Knott will soon recover'. This, alas, was not to
be. At the moment of triumph, as it were, the selfless Bessie's
health declined. She died on 26 March 1879 from 'chronic
dysentery' after a long illness, age twenty-eight.[13] She was buried
in Dundrum cemetery on 28 March.

Knott's determination was unshaken. He presented the fruits
of anatomical research to learned societies and increased his
academic status immeasurably by becoming FRCSI (1880) and
MRCPI (1881) and then taking the MA and MD of Dublin
University. Domestic felicity was regained by his marriage in
1881 to Philippa Balcombe, daughter of a retired army colonel.[14]
She bore him a son and a daughter.

Despite his brilliant record, a place on the staff of a teaching-
hospital eluded him and he applied unsuccessfully for chairs of
anatomy in Dublin, Belfast and Sydney. As if in reaction, his research ceased to have immediate relevance to modern progress and
dealt increasingly with the historical and bizarre. He was a prolific
contributor of articles and reviews to the *Dublin Journal of Medical
Science* and the *Medical Press and Circular*. His wide literary interests
will be discussed later.

A letter in November 1882 from a former fellow student,
Thomas Heazle Parke, a native of Drumsna, County Roscommon,
renewed their friendship. Knott had coached Parke for the army
entrance examination and now the army doctor wrote from
Alexandria to describe his experiences in the Tell el Kebir campaign.[15] Some years later, Parke was medical officer to the Emin
Pasha relief expedition led by H.M. Stanley and crossed Africa,
rediscovering *en route* Ptolemy's 'Mountains of the Moon'.
Finding himself a hero on his return to England, Parke decided
to follow the example of Stanley and A.J. Mounteney-Jephson
and write a book about their arduous journey. He turned to

Knott in 1890 for advice. 'I have [he wrote] a fairly good sized diary of my African experiences and I want to compile a book to come out as soon as I can write it. Would you give me a hand with it as you promised[?]'

Parke expected to make £1000 from the book and offered Knott £200 to write it but it must appear under Parke's name. 'I don't wish you to let anyone know that you are doing the work for me as I want it to appear as my own work entirely.' Knott accepted his terms and, using Parke's notes and diary, wrote *My Personal Experiences in Equatorial Africa*, which was published in 1891. Knott also 'ghosted' Parke's *Guide to Health in Africa* (1893), a chapter 'Hints on health' for a book issued by the Royal Geographical Society, and a number of magazine articles which attracted more rejection slips than acceptances from editors tired of Africa.

Parke, in great demand as a lecturer and reviewer, began to call on Knott to deal with even the least of his literary chores. One feels that before long Knott must have rebelled, had not the unusual partnership been terminated by the army doctor's unexpected death in 1893.

Knott, as already mentioned, reviewed regularly for the *Dublin Journal of Medical Science* and the *Medical Press and Circular*. He contributed at least thirty notices to the latter in 1892 and gave a cordial welcome to John William Moore's *Textbook of the Eruptive and Continued Fevers*.

The author is an ex-scholar (classical), as well as a graduate of Trinity College, Dublin; and the significance of this fact is obvious on every page. He has already won his laurels in the domain of medical literature – in the department of prosody. It has been customary to indicate the quantity of the middle vowel in the term '*angina*' with something like a diminutive spirit level, with the central bubble left out and separated from the upper end of its letter by a gaseous space reminding the reader of Boutigny's researches on the 'spheroidal state' of liquids. Some have, however, endeavoured to show that the quantity should really be marked by a figure like that of a lilliputian boomerang with the concavity turned up. In the pages of this journal some years ago Professor John William Moore proved himself an enthusiastic advocate of the boomerang-shaped quantity, and fortified his arguments with several literary facts furnished by an eminent F.T.C.D.

The editorial departments regarded Knott as careful and reliable and, in a busy moment, the Dublin editor of the *Medical Press and Circular*, Archibald Hamilton Jacob, merely glanced at the opening paragraphs of his critique of a biography of William Stokes. These were conventionally bland but Dr Jacob overlooked Knott's devastating attack on the medical establishment in the tail of the review and read it with horror when printed and circulated. Jacob wrote immediately to scold the errant reviewer:

In the first place such commentary on the profession is not *ad rem* to a review at all. Secondly the language is scurrilous. It is, obviously, a violent attack on certain individuals – any one of whom could maintain a ruinous action for libel to which we could offer no sort of effective defence.

Albert Alfred Tindall, the proprietor and London editor, also expressed regret that Knott's 'review of Stokes had turned out so disastrously for the Journal and Dr Jacob'. He, too, had come to see Knott as 'one of our safest and most impartial reviewers' and had passed the notice without reading it. He went on to say that Jacob had sent him a most temperate letter about the matter. 'He displays no animus, says you are highly capable but indiscreet and says this attack of yours is the most unfortunate thing that has happened for him and for the journal in Dublin.'

T.H. Parke had felt that Dublin was hardly large enough for Knott's talents. He had urged him to establish a link with the *Lancet*, London's leading journal, and eulogized him to its editor. This much-desired connection did not materialize but, early in 1903, Knott was invited to contribute to two transatlantic periodicals, the *New York Medical Journal* and *American Medicine*.

A former acquaintance, Dr Kenneth Millican, who was associate editor of the *New York Medical Journal*, happened to see Knott's article on the Holy Shroud in *Indian Medicine* (edited by J.R. Wallace FRCSI) and wrote on 28 February to enquire 'whether you had forgotten my very existence. I had, of course, not forgotten yours, because I have the testimonial which you once gave me among the things which are always with me.' A week later, pleased with Knott's enthusiastic review of his *Biographic Clinics*, Dr George Milbry Gould, a Philadelphia ophthalmologist and editor of *American Medicine*, penned a letter to that 'best of reviewers' inviting him to become a contributor. 'Good original articles are what we want, containing new and interesting work.' Knott was glad to oblige.

When Millican was appointed editor of a run-down periodical, the *St Louis Medical Review*, in 1904 he implored Knott to send him copy. Knott also wrote for the *St Paul Medical Journal*, the *Medical Record*, the *Canadian Practitioner and Review*, the *Westminster Review* and other journals. Material from his pen in the *Freeman's Journal* is unsigned, in accordance with the rules of the General Medical Council. His reviews, editorials, essays, etc. probably exceeded 2000 in number.

Knott retained an affection for his native county, taking the *Roscommon Herald* regularly, and mentioning in an article on 'touching for "the King's evil"' the 'wavy, hilly-hollow, emerald clad fields of this quiet locality', where he had known the sexton of a parish church close to the Shannon, who had a herbal cure. He was glad to praise colleagues born in County Roscommon: Thomas Heazle Parke, whose career 'was a few years ago so suddenly and sadly terminated in his prime'; Dr Michael Cox,[16] physician to St Vincent's Hospital and 'one of the highest living authorities on Irish history and antiquities'; Oliver Goldsmith, 'one of the brightest ornaments of the world's literature, and of the medical profession'.[17]

Douglas Hyde, born in Castlerea and reared in Frenchpark, had been almost a neighbour of the youth, who lived a few miles up the road at Kingsland. They would have met from time to time in the Royal Irish Academy, of which they were members, and on 13 May 1905, Hyde posted a card from Frenchpark acknowledging an off-print of an article on spontaneous combustion.[18]

A Chara,

A thousand thanks for your intensely interesting study on Sp. Com. I have so often heard of it but never really knew anything about it. Everything you write is so clear and interesting. Excuse this card but I am up to my eyes in work.

Mise An Craoibín

Off-prints of Knott's articles were widely distributed and he corresponded with editors, colleagues, rare-book dealers and others. Having edited some of Knott's manuscripts, George Milbry Gould complained that his eyes were aching: 'Your ink is poor and pale in several, and you write so finely and condensed that deciphering is often straining.' On another occasion Gould wrote more breezily: 'Glad to get your p.c. and wish I would sit down and have a good talk with you. You must be the nicest fellow and friend. Move over to *this* country! You Irishmen do well here, and we like you . . .'.

Father Dinneen sent the following letter:

R.I. Acad

Tuesday

Dear Dr Knott,

Kindly accept a copy of the Irish School Monthly which contains a little article by me. In that article I had the audacity to drag in your knotty name: 'nomen nodosum'. This is a trifling return pro beneficiis tantis tamen, ne 'sordeant tibi munera nostra'[19] et 'veni rebus non aspera *egenis*'[20] even though you be a *jaynus* (genius)

Yours admiringly

Pádraig Ua Duinnín[21]

William Taylor, surgeon to the Meath Hospital, paid him a generous compliment:

Many a time I say to myself there are two men known to me personally whom I could almost worship, one is Mr Wyndham whose equal as a public speaker for diction and poetical expression I have never yet heard, the other is John Knott for the extent of his knowledge in connection with subjects other than those of his own profession and for the facility with which he finds words always so expressive of his meaning.

You seem to be able to make all knowledge your own. I wonder could you communicate the gift to a friend.[22]

His correspondents included Edward Dowden, professor of English literature in TCD, who, on 27 October 1902, wrote from Highfield House, Rathmines: 'I begin to think you are Dr Faustus, or Mephistopheles, or the Wandering Jew or somebody a little demonic; you bring curious learning on all manner of subjects out of your conjuring bag.'

He sent a copy of his paper on angina pectoris to William Osler, professor of medicine at Johns Hopkins Hospital, who duly acknowledged it.

1, West Franklin Street,

Baltimore, Md., Oct. 29th, 1904

Dear Dr Knott:–

Your paper on the angina pectoris interested me very much, particularly what you say as to its rarity in Ireland. It seems a very common disease in this country. I have collected now another long series, and hope next year when I get more leisure in Oxford, where I go in May, to issue the second edition of my lectures on the subject.

Very truly yours,

Wm Osler

Osler was devoted to Sir Thomas Browne, the author of *Religio Medici*, and had an outstanding collection of his works. When Knott sent an off-print of his own article on Browne to Dowden, the latter was delighted. 'Since I was quite a boy Sir Thomas has been one of my favourite writers . . . My earliest copy of *Rel. Med.* is 1645, but I have everything else in first editions including A Letter to a Friend, which Dr Osler calls the rarest of all Browne's works.'

When Osler, by then regius professor of medicine at Oxford University, visited Dublin in 1906, he left a card for Knott at the Shelbourne Hotel: 'So sorry to have missed you – only here for a few hours.' Knott's review of the second edition of *Aequanimitas* refers to the valedictory address at Johns Hopkins University in 1905, in the course of which Osler said that the great advances come from men under forty and referred jocosely to Trollope's novel *The Fixed Period*, which proposed 'the admirable scheme of a college into which at sixty men retired for a year of contemplation before a peaceful departure by chloroform'. One presumes, incidentally, that Osler's remarks on that occasion (reported at face value by the newspapers) explain James Joyce's comment in *Finnegans Wake*, 'the ogry Osler will oxmaul us all'.[23]

Osler thanked Knott for an off-print of his article on Bernard Connor (1666–98), an Irishman who became doctor to the King of Poland. 'Delighted with your Bernard Connor. It is nice that you have done justice in his memory.'

Dowden enjoyed Knott's paper on Dr Thomas Dover (1660–1742), the buccaneer physician who rescued Alexander Selkirk (the model for Robinson Crusoe) from the island of Juan Fernandez. '"Dover" is most interesting [Dowden wrote]. I wish I could supplement it by a sight of Woodes Roger's A Cruising Voyage round the World 1712. If I lecture my College class on Defoe I shall now take care to tell them of Thomas Dover.'

III

From a literary viewpoint, Knott is mainly a purveyor of arcana abstracted from recondite sources and embellished with quotations which would have benefited from editorial pruning. G.M. Gould cautioned him against 'glittering generalities and flowering redundancies'. He had a flair for salty metaphors (his reference, for instance, to a theory 'firmly imbedded in the petrifying cement of the *Transactions of the Royal Society*') and indulged in arresting *obiter dicta* such as ' "Philosophic doubt" has never been a favoured guest in the halls of learned institutions.' His interests, as Widdess indicated, were endless; he wrote with equal enthusiasm on 'the practice of kissing', the odd but universal custom of 'salutation after sneezing' and the plica polonica. Let us consider more closely three of his papers – 'Michael Servetus and the discovery of the circulation of the blood'[24]; 'Sir Walter Raleigh's "Royal Cordial" '[25]; and 'Sir Thomas Browne, Knight, Doctor of Physick . . . Witch-Finder'.[26]

In the first of these, Knott tells how Michael Servetus and John Calvin, who shared 1509 as natal year,[27] were thrown together by fate in Paris and Geneva. Through Calvin's machinations sentence of death was passed on Servetus in 1553 for heresy and the atrabilious theologian gloated over the execution from his bedroom window.

Michael Servetus was slowly roasted at the stake with a small supply of faggots, which was purposely chosen *greenish* in quality (so as to insure slow combustion). He was *crowned* with a straw wreath sprinkled with brimstone – which was *first* fired by the executioner's torch. *Tied to his thigh* was the volume which contained his cherished theological doctrines, and the *first printed description of the circulation of the blood* in the human body.

The clarification of the circulation of the blood is generally credited to William Harvey (*De Motu Cordis*, 1628); he proved experimentally that the heart (a muscular pump) drives blood from its left ventricle into distributing arterial conduits which take it to all tissues, from which it is returned through the veins to the heart's right-sided chambers, whence (after a 'lesser circulation' through the lungs) it reaches left-sided chambers to be driven again from the contracting left ventricle into the arterial channels. Knott unfairly minimizes Harvey's contribution. His plea that since antiquity, 'an approximately accurate conception of the *general* circulation' existed, is ably supported by a familiarity with the ancient texts. He calls witnesses from the schools of Cos and Alexandria, selecting Rabelais as a medieval spokesman:

and through the Veins is sent to all the Members; each Parcel of the Body draws it then into its self, and after its own Fashion is cherished and ailmented by it: Feet, Hands, Thighs, Arms, Eyes, Ears, Back, Breast, yea, all; and thus it is that who before were Lenders, now become *Debtors*.

The brilliance of Michael Servetus's contribution is uncontestable, albeit the existence of a circulation of the blood through the lungs had already been postulated by Ibn an-Nafis in the mid-thirteenth century.[28] But few copies of *Christianismi Restitutio* survived; the discovery by Servetus of the pulmonary circulation remained unknown until 1694 and did not influence William Harvey, the magnitude of whose achievement, a great triumph for experimental medicine, was not fully appreciated by John Knott.

The essay on Raleigh's cordial is as good an example as any of Knott's discursiveness and penchant for lengthy quotations. He leavens his text with yeasty anecdotes such as that of Raleigh's promise to provide Salisbury, a hunchbacked dwarf ('known to have inspired Bacon's *Essay on Deformity*'), with an accommodating virgin but, in the event, the trusting nobleman went to bed to a harlot with the pox, with regrettable consequences; or another on the same indelicate theme concerning a disobliging cuckold who purposefully lay with a French whore in order to pass on her infections to his wife, who, in turn, gave a vile disease to James II, her royal lover, leaving him unequipped for further amorous adventures.

Knott outlines Raleigh's career and travels, describes his introduction to the Court, where he became a favourite of Queen Elizabeth – 'whose susceptibility of heart still retained its apparently vernal freshness, despite its physiological service of nearly half a century' – and refers to his vigorous practice 'of the piracy (for it was no other) which occupied on the "Spanish Main", one of the most active and interesting sections of his chequered career'. He takes us on the cold morning of 29 October 1618 to hear Sir Walter Raleigh's words as he looked at the executioner's axe: 'This gives me no fear. It is a sharp and fair medicine to cure me of all my diseases.'

He supplies an analysis of the cordial which Raleigh elaborated during his incarceration in the Tower of London. Its ingredients included powered hartshorn, dried viper flesh, extract of chermes berries, wood of aloes and sarsaparilla, bezoar stone, magistery of coral, ambergrise and other substances animal, vegetable and mineral, a list such as Huysmans might have featured in *À rebours*. When given to Queen Anne, the cordial arrested her seemingly incurable illness but young Prince Henry took it unavailingly and died on 6 November 1612.

Sir Thomas Browne, the famous author of *Religio Medici*, was born on 19 October 1605. Knott's paper to welcome the approaching tercentenary was published in the *Dublin Journal of Medical Science*. He dismisses as unflattering 'to the physical attractions of women' Browne's fastidious wish that 'we might procreate like trees without conjunction', nor does he show evident approval of Browne's rather self-satisfied expression of male superiority – 'Man is the whole World . . . Woman the Rib and crooked piece of man.' He deals briefly with *Pseudodoxia Epidemica* and Browne's other writings and credits him with 'what may be fairly regarded as a pre-Darwinian suggestion of the influence of climate and environment on animal "complexion"', but he is principally concerned to defend Sir Thomas's belief in witchcraft when seen in proper perspective.

Buttressed by biblical sanction, a belief in witches was almost universal in the seventeenth century and, to Knott's mind, 'Browne's views on this head were the reverse of exceptional; the worst that can justly be said of them is that they display a suspicion of narrow conservatism in some directions, as does his contemptuous rejection of the Copernican system of astronomy.' He will not accuse Sir Thomas of ill-feeling or cruelty towards Amy Duny and Rose Cullender, whose ill-fate was probably determined by his evidence at their trial for witchcraft at Bury St Edmunds in 1665, the last trial of its kind in England. He is more generous than his Dublin colleague, Dr Conolly Norman, Medical Superintendent of the Richmond Asylum, who insisted that Sir Thomas Browne's record is stained with innocent blood. 'The bench had its scruples, but no scruples appear to have troubled the doctor who was ready to sacrifice two helpless victims of popular prejudice, two women whom he should have looked upon as his patients . . .'.[29]

Knott returned to Sir Thomas Browne in a paper published in the *British Medical Journal*.[30] He rebuked Conolly Norman for the 'clumsy sarcasm' with which he treated Browne's reverence for 'the distinct number of three', an indication that Dr Norman really had no conception of the age-old symbolism of numbers such as one, three and seven. Three is a particularly sacred number:

All known things may be said to exist in threes: beginning, middle, and end; past, present and future. Not only is all time thus contained in three, but so, too, is all space: in length, breadth, and thickness – circumscribed within line, surface, and body. God, as the prophet pointed out, orders the world by three: number, weight, and measure. The human microcosm consisted of a trinity: body, soul, and spirit. The soul itself was triple: vegetative, added at the moment of conception; sensitive, at the time of quickening; and intellectual, at the instant of first breathing.

Knott's brilliant summary of the evolution of an intelligible cosmology prior to the dawn of modern science explains how under pressures of good and evil the insights of primitive man entailed a belief in beneficient spirits, baneful demons and witches – pagan ideas still subconsciously nurtured in the minds of the first Christian theologians. Even the élite of the seventeenth century believed in witches and their infernal craft. John Wesley said in the following century that to give up witchcraft was to give up the Bible; Friedrich Hoffmann, 'who may be regarded as the father of the modern theory and practice of medicine', believed in demons; Antonius de Haen, 'the first physician who systematically used the clinical thermometer', published *De Magia* in 1775. 'In presence of such a cloud of witnesses,' Knott asked, 'who can accuse the great Norwich physician of either cruelty or ignorance?'

IV

Once-fashionable York Street underwent a social change resembling those affecting unfortunate families. As the grimy tenements increased in number the professional men departed and the Knotts, caught in the trend, moved in 1910 to 2 Sally-mount Terrace, Ranelagh.

Knott's 'Dublin Letter' in the January 1911 issue of the *St Louis Medical Review* (where it could hardly be of great local interest) shows how little the remonstrances of Jacob and Tindall had influenced him. Again his target is the medical establishment and he foretells that an approaching election of a Master of the Rotunda Hospital 'will be found to give the fullest play to the Tammany Hall tactics which have evermore presided over the elections to professional positions in this country where "friendship" and "job" pervade the whole area of campaign . . .'.

Advancing into his sixties, Knott persisted with his literary endeavours. He accepted a commission from Messrs Baillière, Tindall & Cox to translate into English Eugène Louis Doyen's three-volume *Operative Surgery*. He was to be paid £120 and worked on the project steadily during the second half of 1913, his methods, as we see from their letter, causing the publishers some inconvenience. 'There is no need to send the manuscript in daily dribblets of a few pages, but if you send it week by week it will do quite well.'

Knott's 'A medical man's peep into ante-bellum Russia' appeared in the *Dublin Journal of Medical Science* in 1917. His last publication was possibly 'Montpellier and its mediaeval fame', a letter carried by the *Medical Press and Circular* on 26 May 1920.

John Freeman Knott died in his home on 2 January 1921; the certified cause of death was influenza and heart failure.

NOTES

1. J.B. Lyons, *Scholar and Sceptic* (Dublin 1985), outlines James Henry's career; Wilde's biography, *Victorian Doctor* (London 1942), was written by another paramedical author, T.G. Wilson; F.S. Bourke, physician to Dr Steevens's Hospital, has contributed a handlist of Kirkpatrick's publications to the *Irish Journal of Medical Science* (1954), 371–4; the introduction to William Doolin, *Dublin's Surgeon-Anatomists and Other Essays* (ed. J.B. Lyons) (Dublin 1987), is biographical; Widdess (1906–82) was librarian and professor of biology, RCSI; Patrick Logan, physician to James Connolly Memorial Hospital, wrote *Making the Cure* (Dublin 1972) and other books and articles.

2. *Freeman's Journal, The Irish Times*, 4 January 1921; *Irish Independent*, 5 January 1921; *Irish Independent*, 5 January 1921; *Medical Press and Circular*, 12 January 1921; *Lancet*, 15 January 1921; *Irish Book-Lover*, no. 12 (1921), 117–18.

3. Eleanor Knott (1886–1975) was appointed lecturer in Celtic Languages in Dublin University in 1928 and promoted to a chair in Early Irish eleven years later. She was the first woman to become MRIA. For further information on her see *Ériu*, vol. 6 (1975), 182–5.

4. J.D.H. Widdess, *The Royal College of Surgeons in Ireland and its Medical School 1784–1984* (Dublin 1984), p. 153.

5. James J. O'Neill, *Times Literary Supplement*, 13 January 1921.
6. William Knott, the second and last surviving son of Jack Knott of Derrybeg, County Sligo, died at Kingsland on 16 August 1887 in his ninetieth year. As the Knott papers in the RCSI are not yet fully catalogued, individual references are not given to extracts from the journal, letters, off-prints, etc.
7. William Stoker FRCI was demonstrator of anatomy at the RCSI and lived close to the College at 32 York Street.
8. Andrew Irwin, Ballymore, Boyle, County Roscommon.
9. Dr James Little, physician to the Adelaide Hospital and professor of medicine, RCSI.
10. Sir William Stokes (1839–1900) was a son of Dr William Stokes (1804–78) and grandson of Whitley Stokes (1763–1845).
11. Be that as it may, Sir Charles Cameron's *History of the Royal College of Surgeons in Ireland*, 2nd ed. (Dublin 1916) is a valuable reference work. It was said of Cameron (1830–1921), who was public analyst and city medical officer, that 'he appeared to be a permanent feature of Dublin life'.
12. Edward Dillon Mapother FRCSI was surgeon to St Vincent's Hospital and professor of physiology, RCSI. The third edition of his *Manual of Physiology* was edited by Knott.
13. 'Chronic dysentery' would not be an acceptable diagnosis today; one might consider ulcerative colitis, tuberculous enteritis or a malabsorption syndrome as possible explanations for her death.
14. In 1875 Oscar Wilde was attracted to her sister, Florence, who later married Bram Stoker.
15. Parke's adventures are summarized in J.B. Lyons, *Brief Lives of Irish Doctors* (Dublin 1987), pp. 126–9. The Knott papers contain 170 letters from Parke to Knott.
16. The Rt Hon. Michael Francis Cox (1851–1926), a native of Drumsna, practised medicine in Sligo before gaining an appointment to the staff of St Vincent's Hospital, Dublin. His publications included 'The Country and Kindred of Oliver Goldsmith', *Journal of the National Literary Society of Ireland*, vol. 1 (1900), 81–111 and *Notes of the History of the Irish Horse* (Dublin 1897). He was appointed to the Privy Council in 1911.
17. Oliver Goldsmith's birthplace has been disputed and it has been suggested that he was born at Pallas, County Longford, rather than at Elphin; but see J. J. Kelly, *The Early Haunts of Oliver Goldsmith* (Dublin 1905), *passim*.
18. This astonishing phenomenon, which is used ingeniously by John Banville to dispose of Granny Godkin in *Birchwood*, was named by Charles Dickens in *Bleak House*. Its actual occurrence is verified, as a great rarity, by Professor P. J. Bofin, the City Coroner, who has cited an instance in his own experience in Dublin – during the night of 27 March 1970 an elderly woman burst into flames without apparent cause and her body was reduced to ashes – and knows of a similar death in Leeds and two in Cardiff – see Dick Alstrom, *The Irish Times*, 26 April 1989.
19. Virgil, *Eclogues*, 2, 44.
20. Virgil, *Aeneid*, 9, 365.

21. Rev. Patrick Stephen Dinneen (1860–1934) compiled the first modern Irish-English dictionary (1904).

22. Sir William Taylor (1871–1933), president RCSI in 1916–18 – see J.B. Lyons, *An Assembly of Irish Surgeons* (Dublin 1984), pp. 46–9.

23. James Joyce, *Finnegans Wake* (London 1939), 317.16.

24. *The Medical Record* (9 September 1911).

25. *Dublin Journal of Medical Science*, no. 121 (1906), 63–70, 131–43.

26. *Ibid.*, no. 120 (1905), 241–4.

27. Michael Servetus was probably born in 1511.

28. Ibn an-Nafis described the lesser circulation in the thirteenth century. See Max Myerhof, *Studies in Medieval Arabic Medicine* (London 1984), VI, pp. 100–20.

29. Conolly Norman, 'Sir Thomas Browne: "Audi Alteram Partem"' *British Medical Journal*, no. 474 (1804), 777–8.

30. 'Medicine and Witchcraft in the Days of Sir Thomas Browne', *British Medical Journal*, vol. 2 (1905), 957–61, 1046–9.

7

*The Death of Oscar Wilde: A Post-Mortem**

> *Since the majority of pyogenic affections
> of the brain arise from neglected otitis
> media, they ought to be regarded as
> preventable diseases, and their prophylaxis
> scrupulously attended to.*
> William Macewen (1893)

'What lies before me is my past,' Oscar Wilde observed in *De Profundis*. Critical dissection of that past since 1900 has resulted in his artistic acceptance and moral toleration but uncertainty remains as to why the Irish playwright died in early middle age. Richard Ellmann's recent biography offers neurosyphilis as the cause of death, a diagnosis that hardly accords with the clinical picture which Ellmann himself and others describe.[1] The question merits re-examination, paying due attention to the natural history and pathology of syphilis hitherto neglected by biographers.

FAMILY HISTORY

Oscar Wilde was born at 21 Westland Row, Dublin, on 16 October 1854, the second child of Mr (later Sir) William Wilde, a surgeon specializing in diseases of the ear and eye, and his wife, Jane Francesca Elgee, a poet and writer. The boy's grandfathers were Thomas Wilde, a country doctor, and Charles Elgee, a Wexford solicitor. What little is known of the grandparents has no clinical relevance.

Sir William and Lady Wilde, short and tall respectively, seemed an ill-assorted pair and it has been easier to point to their

*   Reprinted from F.C. Rose (ed.), *Neuroscience across the Centuries* (London 1989), pp. 227–37.

eccentricities than to appreciate their worth. 'Why are Sir William Wilde's nails so black'? asked a wag. The answer: 'Because he scratches himself.' And Lady Wilde was said to have corrected a servant for placing dishes on the coal-scuttle, asking him what chairs were meant for. Oscar's biographers have gloated over every paternal angularity in deterministic explanation of his fall from grace.

The breadth of Sir William Wilde's interests and accomplishments is staggering indeed. His biographer, T.G. Wilson, calls him 'one of the two greatest English-speaking aurists of his time', the other being Joseph Toynbee.[2] He invented many instruments including 'Wilde's snare'; 'Wilde's incision' and 'Wilde's ointment' are the eponyms he earned. He founded St Mark's Ophthalmic Hospital and was Oculist-in-Ordinary to the Queen. He was the author of *Practical Observations on Aural Surgery* and editor of the *Dublin Journal of Medical Science*. Sir Peter Froggatt[3] has published a detailed study of Wilde's work as Assistant Census Commissioner. Colm Ó Lochlainn (1949) called him, 'The first, and still the greatest of our scientific archaeologists.'[4] These accomplishments may have greater relevance to his son's career than his sexual peccadilloes.

Prior to her marriage, using the *nom de plume* 'Speranza', Jane Elgee contributed patriotic verses and articles to *The Nation*. One of her prose pieces, 'Jacta alea est – the die is cast', published on 29 July 1848, led to the newspaper's suppression. Later she established a literary salon at 1 Merrion Square and when living in reduced circumstances in London after her husband's death she still maintained her literary connections. A modern critic, Robert Hogan, has described her Irish folktales as 'absolutely enchanting'.[5]

The elder son, Willie, a bright youngster, read for the bar and later followed journalism in London. Isola, the only daughter, died on 23 January 1867 in her ninth year. She was staying with her aunt at the Glebe, Edgeworthstown, when she died, which suggests that she succumbed to one or other of the many acute infections then prevalent.

Sir William Wilde is believed to have had at least three natural children. These were Dr Henry Wilson (whom the Wilde boys spoke of as their cousin) and two girls, Emily and Mary, who were given their father's surname. They lived in County Monaghan with their uncle, the Reverend Ralph Wilde, and at twenty-four and twenty-two respectively were the victims of a tragic accident when in November 1871 Emily's dress caught fire at a ball. Her sister rushed to help her and Mary's dress was also enveloped by flames. They died from burns.

This extra family of illegitimates is often cited to indicate the father's promiscuous and passionate heterosexual nature. Be that as it may, the close association maintained with Henry Wilson, who qualified LRCSI in 1858 when he was twenty and became an assistant at St Mark's Hospital, and Ralph Wilde's willingness to shelter Emily and Mary (the elder girl named for her paternal grandmother, Emily Fynne), suggest that William Wilde's amours may have been less than sordid. He was most unlikely to have been the 'runner after girls, with a lusty enjoyment of life' portrayed by Arthur Ransome, Oscar Wilde's first biographer.[6]

As Henry Wilson was born in 1838, his putative father would then have been in his early twenties, a recent graduate from the Schools of Surgery and a good matrimonial 'catch'. He accompanied a wealthy invalid on a health cruise, as personal doctor, and was away from Ireland from September 1837 to June 1838. Dr Robert Graves is said to have sent young Wilde abroad to improve his health, but a more urgent reason for his departure may have been the need to escape from a designing lady who was left, literally, holding the baby.

The libel action taken against Lady Wilde by Mary Josephine Travers had Sir William as its target. The doctor had certainly been tactless and foolish in making so much of his young patient and then cooling their relationship, but it is unlikely that he ravished her or that she deserved more than the derisory farthing damages. The pitfalls of biography, incidentally, are nicely illustrated by the following cautionary tale.

On the evidence of one of Miss Travers's letters to Wilde quoted in the account of the trial carried by *Saunders Newsletter*, which reported her promise 'to take up your son as soon as ever I can', T.G. Wilson understandably concluded that Wilde had had a sexual affair with the girl, who bore him a son.[7] But by consulting other newspapers, Terence de Vere White detected the *Newsletter*'s extraordinary misprint. Miss Travers had actually promised 'to take up your I.O.U.'. That 'desperately serious error', as de Vere White has pointed out, 'has been used as evidence of Wilde's profligacy'.[8]

Sir William Wilde completed his *Report of the 1871 Census* in 1874 but towards the end of the following year his health declined and 1876 failed to bring the hoped-for recovery. He died on 19 April 1876 and the progressive asthenia suggests that he died from cancer.

He was succeeded as Senior Surgeon to St Mark's Hospital by Henry Wilson FRCSI, author of *Lectures on the Theory and Practice of the Ophthalmoscope* (1868), whose tenure of the post was brief. Wilson attended a meeting of the Board of Governors on 28 May 1877. He missed a special meeting on 11 June because of illness but sent a rough draft of his report for 1876. Two days later he was dead. He was unmarried and left £1000 and £250 to his 'cousins' Willie and Oscar Wilde respectively but disappointed them by leaving the bulk of his fortune to the hospital, £4000.[9]

Lady Wilde died on 3 February 1896. She had suffered from bronchitis and the precise cause of her death is unknown. Willie Wilde's death on 13 March 1899 has been attributed to alcoholism and did not surprise Oscar, whose comment to a friend was, 'I suppose it had been expected for some time . . . Between him and me there had been, as you know, wide chasms for many years. *Requiescat in pace*.'[10]

Whether or not Oscar himself escapes a diagnosis of alcoholism is, as we shall see, debatable but, other than disclosure of a trait shared by the brothers, a scrutiny of the family's medical history is negative for relevant clinical data. The emerging positive fact is that the father was an 'over-achiever', the mother similarly gifted, their union a likely source of liberally endowed offspring.

SOCIAL HISTORY

At Portora School near Enniskillen, Oscar Wilde was regarded as less able than his brother, nor did he shine at games, saying that he 'never liked to kick or be kicked'. At Dublin University and Magdalen College, Oxford, where he held scholarships, his intellectual brilliance was evident and his forceful, irreverent personality and cultivation of the beautiful attracted puzzled attention.

Although caricatured as a silly aesthete by Gilbert and Sullivan in *Patience*, he was tall and powerfully built. A sportsman in early manhood, he enjoyed himself in Connemara in the summer of 1877. 'The fishing has not been so good as usual,' he reported to a friend. 'I only got one salmon, about 7½lbs. The sea trout however are very plentiful . . .'. The evenings were devoted to 'Pool, Ecarté and Potheen Punch' and he broke the journey to Dublin to shoot partridge in Longford. He was responsive to feminine allure and boasted in a letter from Dublin (6 August 1876) that he was taking a delightful girl to service in the Cathedral. This was Florence Balcombe, his first love, whom he might have married had she been other than the daughter of a retired army officer and lacking a private income.

Wilde's powerful frame and his mother's large, ungainly figure led George Bernard Shaw to say that Oscar and Speranza were examples of pituitary gigantism. This absurdity is more understandable when it is recalled that Pierre Marie's description of acromegaly (1886) and D.J. Cunningham's demonstration that Cornelius Magrath, the Irish giant, had a pituitary gland lesion, had made pituitary disorders fashionable.[11] Shaw's comment was rejected by T.G. Wilson who, nevertheless, spoke of Oscar as 'a pituitary type', invoking a non-existent physiological concept. James Joyce's reference to the 'epileptic tendency' of Wilde's nervous system was equally inept.[12] Nor is homosexuality to be facilely explained on a detail like the use of female apparel as a toddler.

There are grounds for believing that Wilde contracted syphilis from a female prostitute at Oxford and that treatment with mercury blackened his teeth.[13] Apart from this his health was good and in 1884 he married Constance Lloyd, a pretty and amiable girl, with some private means, who was to bear him two unblemished sons. He was deeply in love with his bride and, meeting a friend in Paris during the honeymoon, he said marriage was wonderful and expatiated in an embarrassing way on their physical raptures. Within a few years, however, he was seeking male lovers. His first homosexual affair began in 1888, initiated by seventeen-year-old Robert Ross. Lionel Johnson introduced him in 1891 to Lord Alfred Douglas, who caused his downfall. But by then he was consorting promiscuously with male prostitutes and sybaritic living had led to a measure of obesity.

Within a decade he attained the culmination of his fame and notoriety. *The Importance of Being Earnest* was playing to full houses but nemesis in the frantic form of the Marquess of Queensberry, father of Lord Alfred Douglas, was prowling outside the theatre.

Lacking that element of self-preservation that had protected Sir William Wilde from interrogation by Miss Travers's lawyers, Oscar's psychopathic egoism impelled him to charge the Marquess of Queensberry with criminal libel only to end up in the dock himself. Some of his young associates appeared at the Old Bailey as prosecution witnesses. They spoke unblushingly of mutual masturbation, sodomy and oral sex.[14] Wilde was sentenced to two years' imprisonment with hard labour.

CLINICAL PICTURE

'Sins of the flesh are nothing,' Wilde wrote in *De Profundis*. 'They are maladies for physicians to cure, if they should be cured.' His correspondence (Wilde, 1962) contains few health references. 'I am very wretched and ill,' he told a friend in March 1878, 'and as soon as possible I am to be sent somewhere out of Oxford.' He convalesced in Bournemouth at the Royal Bath Hotel. During the American tour he referred to a minor upset when writing to Samuel Ward, elder brother of Julia Ward Howe, author of 'The Battle Hymn of the Republic': 'I am much better – feel well and happy – very little pain of any kind: slept well also. You are a magician, and a master of all things from finance to a dinner, from lyrics to medicine . . .'. There was 'a severe attack of asthma' in 1885 and an ill-defined indisposition towards the end of February 1891. Constance Wilde told her brother on 7 July 1892 that Oscar was at Bad-Homburg for a rest-cure, 'getting up at 7.30, going to bed at 10.30, smoking hardly any cigarettes and being massaged, and of course drinking waters'. A letter from Wilde to Rothenstein, the artist, ends plaintively: 'I am very ill, dear Will, and can't write any more.' Two years later he was laid up briefly with what he called 'a sort of malarial fever' but was probably influenza.

The health record assembled from his early letters is that of infrequent, commonplace indispositions but, as already mentioned, biographers say that he contracted syphilis at Oxford. Ellmann suggests, on the dubious evidence of a bookseller's catalogue, that Wilde addressed the poem 'Taedium Vitae' to the whore who infected him.[15]

Evidently Wilde made the initial recovery to be expected in primary lesions. He sought medical advice before proposing to Constance and was assured that 'cure' was effected (Montgomery Hyde, 1976). 'About two years later he discovered to his dismay that all traces of syphilis had not been eradicated from his system; on the contrary the spirochaetes were quite active.'[16] The validity of this somewhat anachronistic statement by Montgomery Hyde (the causative germ was not isolated until 1905), based on some 'unpublished and unpublishable letters' of Robert Sherard to A.J.A. Symons, is difficult to assess. But the examinations by prison doctors familiar with the repertoire of syphilis evidently disclosed no further lesions. Wilde had no good word, incidentally, for the prison MOs. 'They are as a class ignorant men. The pathology of the mind is unknown to them.' 'As a class they are brutes, and excessively cruel.'

'For myself, I am ill and apathetic,' Wilde wrote from Holloway Jail. 'Slowly life creeps out of me.' Apart from loss of freedom and the personal indignities of prison life, he suffered from lack of edible food, diarrhoea, and insomnia, aggravated by the plank bed. On 8 March 1897, however, he assured a friend, More Adey, that he was free of organic disease though, in saying so, he forgot the 'running ear' mentioned in his petition to the Home Secretary on 2 July 1896. He had 'almost entirely lost the hearing of his right ear through an abscess that had caused a perforation of the drum'. The medical officer was unable to help and predicted complete loss of hearing in the affected ear (which had been worsened when Wilde fainted and fell in the prison chapel) whereas he had been assured by Sir William Dalby FRCS, a leading London aurist, that with proper care hearing should be retained. Wilde's second petition on 10 November 1896 conceded that his ear was 'attended to daily'. There was no relief, however, from the 'terrible mental stress and anguish' which he feared would lead to insanity and the refusal to commute his sentence was 'like a blow from a leaden sword'.

'I quiver in every nerve with pain,' he told More Adey. 'I am wrecked with the recurring tide of hysteria. I can't sleep. I can't eat.' Through this dreadful annealing he did attain positive gains:

'I have no bitterness at all', he told Michael Davitt after his release, 'but I have learnt pity: and that is worth learning, if one has to tramp a yard for two years to learn it.' He spent his remaining years in France with occasional visits to Italy and Switzerland, his existence determined by a need for economies which he consistently circumvented, and by an element of fatalism. 'One of the many lessons that one learns in prison is that things are what they are, and will be what they will be.'

In his petitions to the Home Secretary, with the hope of clemency, Wilde referred to his offences as 'forms of sexual madness . . . diseases to be cured by a physician, rather than crimes to be punished by a judge'. Fundamentally he was unchanged and unrepentant: 'A patriot put in prison for loving his country', he reasoned, 'loves his country, and a poet in prison for loving boys loves boys.' He also drank heavily, preferring brandy and absinthe. 'I hear that he does nothing now but drink,' his wife (who had changed her name to Holland) remarked to a mutual friend, and Edouard Dupoirier, the generous *patron* of Wilde's main base in Paris, the Hôtel d'Alsace, indicated that he drank more than a litre of brandy daily.

He was distressed to learn in July 1897 that Constance had a spinal complaint causing pain and paralysis. Her increasing agony led to an operation in a Genoa hospital but she died a few days later on 7 April 1898. Montgomery Hyde and Ellmann relate her misfortune, unconvincingly, to a previous accident. She had tripped over a loose stair rod in her London home, falling down a flight of stairs and injuring her back. One recalls that Captain Gilbey, whose meningioma Victor Horsley removed in the first successful operation of its kind on 10 June 1887, had experienced trauma which delayed diagnosis.[17]

The emergence of progressive pain and paralysis some years after recovery from the fall suggests recent compressive disease, benign or malignant, and carries no suspicion of a lesion acquired from her husband. A decade had elapsed since Horsley had cured Gilbey's paraplegia but spinal surgery was still at an early stage; X-rays had only just become available and mortality rates were high. When Wilde visited Constance's grave in Genoa, he felt regret but realized the futility of regret. 'Nothing could have been otherwise, and Life is a very terrible thing.'

Writing from a café on 8 May 1898, he described a recent throat operation, the exact nature of which is unknown. 'The operation itself was all right, as I was drenched with cocaine, but afterwards it was very painful . . .'.

'I should go and see my doctor today,' he wrote to Reginald Turner a few days later, 'but I don't like to, as I am not feeling very well. I only care to see doctors when I am in perfect health; then they comfort one, but when one is ill they are most depressing.'

A doctor in Nice treating his gout in February 1899 put him off champagne but, with the expectation of unlimited quantities of his favourite wine at a friend's house in Switzerland, Wilde had little intention of complying. During November and December of that year and the early part of 1900 he felt unwell and unable to rise before afternoon.

His throat bothered him again in February 1900. He mentioned a disease 'with a hybrid-Greek name' to Leonard Smithers, publisher of *The Ballad of Reading Gaol*: 'it attacks the throat and the soul'. 'I am very ill . . .', he told Robert Ross. 'My throat is a lime kiln, my brain a furnace and my nerves a coil of angry adders.' He spent ten days in hospital and had recovered by March though still affected by a rash: 'and when one has one's bath one looks like a leopard'.

This illness was ascribed to mussel-poisoning but in Ellmann's account the rash – 'great red splotches on his arms, chest and back' – first occurred in the summer of 1899.[18] It was intensely itchy and, according to Wilde's February letter, 'very painful'. Unexpectedly, almost 'miraculously', he was cured of the 'mussel-poisoning' at Easter, having received the Pope's blessing in the Vatican.

He had an eerie experience in Rome. Whenever he passed his hotel, which he did frequently, he saw the same man go by. 'Scientists call the phenomenon an obsession of the optic nerve,' he told Ross. 'You and I know better.' Macdonald Critchley (1957) interprets this episode as an example of 'visual perseveration', which occasionally occurs in parieto-occipital lesions or mild delirium.[19] One might also see it as distantly related to autoscopic hallucination.[20] Fortunately there was no recurrence. Was it just a figment of the playwright's lively imagination? It is important to stress that Wilde's intellectual faculties and capacity to amuse were intact until the last days of an acute illness. This fact, together with the absence of convulsions or apoplectiform episodes, rules out general paralysis of the insane (GPI).

The rash reappeared. A doctor in Paris put it down to neurasthenia and Wilde was well enough to visit Switzerland in August.

On his return to Paris his correspondence was mainly directed to raising funds. His habitual needs were increased by an exacerbation of his ear complaint, for which he consulted Dr Maurice a'Court Tucker, a general practitioner favoured by the English colony.

'The operation I have had to undergo [in the hotel on 10 October] was a most terrible one,' he told Frank Harris. 'The surgeon's fee is 1500 francs (£60) . . . I also have to have a hospital male nurse all day, and a doctor to sleep at night in the room. I then have to pay my own doctor, who comes daily, and the hotel for another room; and the chemist's bill is about £20 already.' Morphine, chloral hydrate and opium were favoured anodynes.

When Robert Ross came to see him on 17 October Wilde said the pain was dreadful but he was in good spirits, laughing and telling stories against the doctors and himself. Visiting him daily, Ross found him talkative and, though he looked ill, capable of amusing his friends with quips such as the well-known 'I am dying beyond my means.' Getting up on 29 October for the first time in some weeks, Wilde went to a café in the evening and drank absinthe. Next day he had a 'cold' and an increased earache but Dr Tucker permitted a drive in the *Bois*.

The male nurse or *panseur*, Hennion, warned Ross that Wilde was gravely ill and would not live more than a few months if he did not change his ways. He hinted that Tucker did not realize the seriousness of the situation and that the ear trouble was really not of much importance. But when Ross spoke to Tucker, the doctor implied that Wilde was better and insisted on having the patient's permission before discussing his case fully. Ross and Tucker met a few days later; the doctor was vague, inclined to claim improvement but agreeing with Hennion that Wilde would die if he continued to drink. The interview upset Wilde, who knew they were discussing his future, or lack of it. He told Ross and Reggie Turner gloomily that he dreamt that he had been supping with the dead. 'My dear Oscar,' Turner said, 'you were probably the life and soul of the party.' Wilde's spirits were immediately restored.

When Ross called on 12 November before joining his mother on the Riviera, Wilde walked about the room talking volubly and emotionally. During the following week he drove in the *Bois* with Turner and seemed better. He dictated a long letter to Frank Harris, another plea for money, completing it in his own hand. On 25 November he felt giddy and stayed in bed. Fever, headache and disorientation followed. His mind wandered in two languages and the clinical picture indicated spread of infection intra-cranially from the middle ear. The doctor sought a second opinion and the following bulletin (translated by Richard Ellmann) was issued on 27 November by Dr Paul Cleiss and Dr Tucker:

The undersigned doctors, having examined Mr Oscar Wilde . . . on Sunday 15 November, established that there were significant cerebral disturbances stemming from an old suppuration of the right ear, under treatment for several years.

On the 27th, the symptoms became much graver. The diagnosis of encephalitic meningitis must be made without doubt. In the absence of any indication of localization, trepanning cannot be contemplated. The treatment advised is purely medicinal. Surgical intervention seems impossible.[21]

Wilde's condition continued to deteriorate; aphasia developed and he died on 30 November 1900 at 1.50 p.m.

DIFFERENTIAL DIAGNOSIS

Biographers generally pass hurriedly over the processes of birth and dying, having had few, if any, opportunities to observe either phenomenon. Ellmann, however, dwells in lurid detail on Wilde's painful passing: 'He had scarcely breathed his last when the body exploded with fluids from the ear, nose, mouth and other orifices.'[22] The diagnosis he offers is neurosyphilis and it is to be hoped that non-medical readers are not misled into regarding as intrinsic to the clinical picture those agonal and post-agonal occurrences – the terminal pulmonary oedema and the unpleasant discharges contingent on relaxed sphincters which distressed Oscar's friends. The diagnosis, moreover, is patently incorrect. Wilde's doctors have stated plainly that the meningo-encephalitis resulted from chronic aural suppuration.

Elsewhere in the biography, Ellmann remarks that opinion is divided and that the 'evidence is not decisive' but I submit that this is not so. There are overwhelming arguments against a diagnosis of neurosyphilis based on its natural history and pathology, whereas the clinical picture might, indeed, be cited as a classical instance of intra-cranial suppuration.

Natural History of Syphilis

Syphilis has been spoken of as 'a fever divided by time'; its clinical features fall into three groups, *primary*, *secondary* and *tertiary* but more than 60 per cent of infected persons escape tertiary manifestations though untreated and about 30 per cent achieve spontaneous cure.[23] It was, therefore, by no means inevitable that sooner or later Wilde must pay for his youthful folly. His concerned friends, Ross and Turner, might not have known this.

Neurosyphilis occurs in less than 10 per cent of persons infected with the *Treponema pallidum* according to Lord Brain[24] – the figure given by Csonka is 4 per cent – and if Ellmann asserts, as he appears to, that Wilde died from acute syphilitic meningitis, it may be pointed out that this is an uncommon condition with a good prognosis and occurs within a year or two of infection.[25] Cases of tertiary neurosyphilis, to which Turner attributed Wilde's demise, may be placed in two main groups: *meningo-vascular* and *parenchymatous* (*tabes dorsalis* and *GPI*) but as this classification will mean little to the reader untutored in pathology, examples may be cited – Charles Baudelaire's aphasia and hemiplegia (meningo-vascular syphilis); Guy de Maupassant's madness (GPI); Karen Blixen's gastric crises and lightning pains (tabes dorsalis). The manifestations of neurosyphilis are protean but with patterns rather different from the acute, devastating complications of bacterial infections of the middle ear.

Pathology of Syphilis

The plasma cell is the hallmark of tertiary syphilis, which causes necrosis and atrophy rather than suppuration. Absence of secondary infection is a characteristic of tertiary syphilitic lesions and it is a stated principle that a secondarily infected lesion in a person known to have syphilis may have a separate cause. We have no microscopic data in Wilde's case but a running ear and a perforated ear-drum are typical of the chronic pyogenic infections so common before the availability of antibiotics. Had the aural lesion been anything out of the ordinary one may presume that Sir William Dalby would have detected it and given a more cautious prognosis. Syphilitic lesions of the auditory nerve lead to loss of hearing.

CLINICAL FEATURES

Having considered the clinical features, Macdonald Critchley, a leading London neurologist, concluded that the most plausible explanations were either septic otitis media or syphilis.[26] His support for the latter had diminished when he replied (1958)[27] to A. Hoffer (1957)[28] and recently (1988) he expressed full acceptance of a diagnosis of septic infection.[29] Critchley referred to three kinds of mussel-poisoning, none of which is associated with a chronic skin rash. Details of Wilde's rash are insufficient to permit firm diagnosis. Ellmann agrees that itchiness makes syphilis unlikely. The typical skin lesions of late syphilis (other than the gumma) are nodular, reddish-brown or copper-coloured with a circinate or serpiginous pattern familiar to practitioners in the 1890s.[30]

The edition of Wilde's informative letters was not available when a paper was presented to the Royal Society of Medicine (1958) by Sir Terence Cawthorne FRCS, who concluded that the cause of death was 'an intra-cranial complication of suppurative otitis media'. He speculated (incorrectly) that the left ear was affected and saw the aphasia as a focal sign indicative of 'a temporal lobe abscess in the dominant hemisphere'.[31] With the evidence of an infected *right* ear before them, the attending doctors knew that aphasia was not a localizing sign. The significant sentence in their report, '*En l'absence de tout indice de localisation on ne peut songer à une trépanation,*' shows how they were thinking and that Wilde's illness received informed attention.[32] Robert Ross's strictures were undeserved.

It may be recalled that Durante had successfully removed 35-year-old Chiera Batistelli's left frontal tumour on 1 June 1885. Sir William Macewen's paper, 'Intra-cranial lesions – illustrating some points in connection with the localization of cerebral affections, and the advantage of antiseptic trephining' (*Lancet*, 1881) was followed by his communication in Glasgow to the British Medical Association's Annual Meeting in 1888. Then, in 1893, Macewen 'fairly shook the medical world', to quote Sir Geoffrey Jefferson[33], with his monograph, *Pyogenic Diseases of the Brain and Spinal Cord*.

H. Montgomery Hyde did not demur from Cawthorne's conclusion. Ellmann accepted the surgeon's suggestion that the operation in October could have been either parcentesis of the ear-drum or removal of polyps but failed to record Cawthorne's belief that the playwright 'had been submitted to the then fashionable Wilde's incision for mastoid infection'. The biographer proceeded to offer a diagnosis of syphilis, giving no reason for his rejection of the ear specialist's viewpoint.

Expressing the conviction earlier in the biography that Wilde had syphilis (which may well have been correct regarding the primary stage), Ellmann added: 'that conviction is central to my conception of Wilde's character and my interpretation of many things in his later life'.[34] The legitimate exuberance of creative biography outstrips the restrained pace of pathography. Any intention of attributing a positive influence to syphilis in Wilde's career should, however, be countered by the observation that the disease generally has destructive effects. Claims to the contrary are recorded (Podolsky, 1946, 1955; Fraser, 1981) but, if valid, such instances are exceptional.[35] The evaporation of Wilde's creativity probably relates to the psychological shock of imprisonment, residence abroad and the damaging effects of alcohol.

DIAGNOSIS

Returning to the Hôtel d'Alsace in those sad November days, one finds Hennion, the *panseur*, taking Ross aside and insisting that drink is the enemy. Ross pressed Tucker for information and left for the Riviera convinced that Wilde would rally. The scene is a common one: the nurse, closer to the patient than any other, knew instinctively that Wilde would die but his knowledge of pathology was faulty; the doctor focused his attention anxiously on the potentially lethal ear infection, unprepared for the present to take a stand on alcohol; the bewildered friends,

Ross and Turner, discouraged by the doctor's apparent ineffectuality – Ross called him 'a silly, kind, excellent man' – put their heads together and decided that the actual cause was being overlooked.

Whether the doctors can have given tacit assent to the despairing suggestion that the illness was a ghastly resurrection of the infection acquired at Oxford is conjectural. It is not reflected in their report but evidently gained spurious authority when whispered in literary circles. 'His death . . .', Arthur Ransome (1912) wrote in an account devoid of any appreciation of the nuances of differential diagnosis, 'was directly due to meningitis, the legacy of an attack of tertiary syphilis.'[36] 'The ear trouble . . .', Reginald Turner wrote to Robert Sherard in 1934, 'was only shortly before his death recognized as a tertiary symptom of an infection he had contracted when he was 20.'[37]

Richard Ellmann was unduly influenced by their unwarranted statements which run contrary to the evidence, as I believe I have shown, and should be discounted. The legendary depredations of the *Treponema pallidum* are not exaggerated but syphilis did not topple Oscar Wilde, a victim in all probability of more brutally lethal pyogenic cocci. By one of the recurring ironies of medical history, the Dublin aurist's son died of a complication within the field of his father's endeavours.

CONCLUSION

There is no convincing evidence that Oscar Wilde had tertiary syphilis. A chronic infection of the right ear antedated his imprisonment. An intra-cranial complication – pyogenic meningitis – led to his death following an acute illness on 30 November 1900.

NOTES

1. Richard Ellmann, *Oscar Wilde* (London 1987), *passim*.
2. T.G. Wilson, *Victorian Doctor* (London 1942), *passim*.
3. P. Froggatt, Sir William Wilde and the 1851 census of Ireland, *Med. Hist.* (1965), 9: 302–27.
4. Colm Ó Lochlainn in Foreword to *The Boyne and the Blackwater* by W.R. Wilde (Dublin 1949).
5. Robert Hogan, *Dictionary of Irish Literature* (London 1979), p. 686.

6. Arthur Ransome, *Oscar Wilde* (London 1912), p. 199.

7. Wilson, *op. cit.*, p. 267.

8. Terence de Vere White, *The Parents of Oscar Wilde* (London 1967), p. 182.

9. J. McAuliffe Curtin, 'Henry Wilson, F.R.C.S.I.' *Irish Journal of Medical Science* (1969), 2: 369–78.

10. Rupert Hart-Davis (ed.), *The Letters of Oscar Wilde* (London 1962).

11. V.C. Medvei, *A History of Endocrinology* (Boston 1982), pp. 305–13.

12. Ellsworth Mason and Richard Ellmann, *The Critical Writings of James Joyce* (London 1959), p. 203.

13. H. Montgomery Hyde, *Oscar Wilde* (London 1976), p. 181; Ellmann, *op. cit.*, p. 89.

14. Hyde, *op. cit.*, pp. 237–8.

15. Ellmann, *op. cit.*, p. 89.

16. Hyde, *op. cit.*, p. 184.

17. J.B. Lyons, *The Citizen Surgeon* (London 1966), pp. 50–5.

18. Ellmann, *op. cit.*, p. 544.

19. Macdonald Critchley, 'Oscar Wilde – A Medical Appreciation', *Med. Hist.* (1957), 1: 199–210.

20. Kenneth Dewhurst, 'Autoscopic Hallucinations', *Irish Journal of Medical Science* (1954), 263–7.

21. Ellmann, *op. cit.*, p. 547.

22. *Ibid.*, p. 549.

23. G.W. Csonka in D.J. Weatherall (ed.),*Oxford Textbook of Medicine* (Oxford 1983), pp. 5, 279; A. Heyman in T.H. Harrison (ed.), *Principles of Internal Medicine* (New York 1970), p. 887.

24. W.R. Brain, *Diseases of the Nervous System*, 6th ed. (Oxford 1969), p. 404.

25. H.H. Merritt, *A Textbook of Neurology*, 3rd ed. (London 1963), p. 125.

26. Critchley, *op. cit.*, p. 127.

27. Critchley, 'Oscar Wilde', *Am. J. Psychiat.*, (1958), 114.

28. A. Hoffer, 'Oscar Wilde', *ibid.* (1957), 113: 176–7.

29. Critchley, 'The Death of Oscar Wilde', *British Medical Journal* (1988), 1: 296.

30. A.E.W. McLachlan, *Handbook of Venereal Diseases*, 3rd ed. (Edinburgh 1947), p. 111.

31. Terence Cawthorne, 'The Last Illness of Oscar Wilde', *Proc. Roy. Soc. Med.* (1959), 52: 123–7.

32. Ellmann, *op. cit.*, p. 549.

33. G. Jefferson, *Sir William Macewen's Contributions to Neurosurgery* (Glasgow 1950), p. 26.

34. Ellmann, *op. cit.*, p. 88 fn.

35. See E. Podolsky, 'Genius, Alcohol, Toxins and Lues', *Medical Press* (1955), 28 December, 613–15; Sir Ian Fraser, 'General Paralysis of the Insane', *British Medical Journal* (1981), 283: 1631–2.

36. Ransome, *op. cit.*, p. 199.

37. MS. University of Reading; Reginald Turner's letter, 3 January 1934.

8

Etude Morbide: *The Illness of John Millington Synge*

WALKING in the Luxembourg Gardens, John Millington Synge saw that the lilacs had withered after a day of rain. 'Do flowers mourn like women for their briefness?' he asked. 'In the Luxembourg I see also girls from eighteen to twenty in the blossom of their health, and women with a few babies who are withered.' Nature is cruel to the animate. Crystals and rubies remain eternally beautiful whereas 'women and flowers and artists fulfil their swift task of propagation and pass in a day'.[1]

Synge's own progeny were creations of the mind – verses, articles and plays now accepted as masterpieces of dramatic art. His proposal of marriage to Cherrie Matheson in 1896 was turned down. His romance with Molly Allgood (the actress Máire O'Neill), with whom he fell in love in 1905, progressed favourably but their union was prevented by his declining health.

He was a victim of Hodgkin's disease and it was in connection with this illness that he reported to a private hospital at 10 p.m. on a Friday evening in December 1897. He was given instructions by Nurse Smith. 'I was to be in bed before midnight when a night nurse would come round and bandage my neck – '. Left alone he looked about the room 'peering into cupboards and presses half dreading to unearth the debris of mutilated victims'. He attempted to read Spinoza's ethics but could not concentrate.[2]

The operation was scheduled for midday. During the course of the morning he slipped back into his room to find it prepared for surgery. 'Every available table was covered with enamelled hardware showing many fantastic shapes whose use I was yet to learn. Strange bottles stood in groups beside articles I had never seen even in the windows of surgical outfitters.'[3] When he was taken down to the room at midday three doctors had arrived. Nurse Smith was also there with two younger nurses. Their seriousness irritated him. 'They thought proper to treat me with the misplaced and abominable sympathy we show to young widows and their like.' His attempts to joke misfired. He undressed without the embarrassment he might ordinarily experience if obliged to disrobe in the presence of young women.

The induction of anaesthesia was an unpleasant experience. Eventually 'clouds of luminous mist were swirling round me', and he had the delusion that the doctors were mocking him. 'I'm an initiated mystic,' he yelled, 'I could rend the ground work of your souls . . .'. The clouds rolled over him, opaque and heavy.

I seemed to traverse whole epochs of desolation and bliss. All secrets were open before me, and simple as the universe to its God. Now and then something recalled my physical life, and I smiled at what seemed a moment of sickly infancy. At other time I felt I might return to earth, and laughed aloud to think what a god I should be among men. For there could be no more terror in my life. I was a light, a joy.[4]

Reminders of mundane existence were few and distant – 'for the rest I was in raptures I have no power to translate'. But clouds re-enveloped him; joy receded and as if in a nightmare he became dimly aware of the operation and of his motionless body. Dismayed, he attempted to re-create the ethereal visions. 'I was sick . . . and people were attending me.' A nurse bent over him. 'Are you coming to? It was very satisfactory.'

Her assurance hardly pleased him, intent on fugitive dreams. 'D — the operation . . . If I could only remember, I'd write books, upon books, I'd teach all earth of delight.' He concentrated instead, with absurd and almost drunken pleasure, on regaining control of his body. 'There goes one leg. There's the other. There's one hand. There's the other.' His language was unparliamentary when he could not raise his head.[5]

Next day, Synge felt weak and was content 'to lie still and be talked to . . .'. The doctors looked in during the forenoon. They had thrown aside their gravity now that the ordeal was over and were 'as jovial as one could desire'. Visitors came in the afternoon. By five he was drowsy and the light was lowered. The voices of Sunday strollers and the sound of the trams in Lower

Mount Street were faintly audible. He listened keenly to those distant tokens of a restored environment. 'The impression was very strong on me that I had died the preceding day and come again to life, and this impression has never changed.'[6]

Synge's manuscripts include fragments of an unpublished novel about nurses:

The end of an October evening was fading over the broad low-lying grave-yard of Dinton . . . At one grave only a living figure could be seen where a young girl in nurses uniform knelt or rather crouched upon the 'ground. A plain slab before her bore the inscription Kathleen Steinhart and the hand-kerchief which had dropped unheeded among the rustling leaves was marked at the edge Rachel Steinhart for the two were twins.[7]

These undeveloped pieces, so different from his acclaimed work, are unequivocal expressions of the influence on Synge's writing of the ill-health that plagued him right through his life. His first memory was of sitting on his nurse's knee while she dressed him at the age of two. 'My promotion to knicker-bockers and a severe cough and croup came about the time that I began to remember coherently.' His childhood 'was a long series of coughs and colds with plenty of amusement in the intervals and summer visits to the sea-side which were delightful'.[8] The Synges were not given to organized games but were energetic walkers and cyclists.

The youngest in a family of eight, he was born on 16 April 1871 at 2 Newton Villas, Rathfarnham, and grew up in Orwell Park, Rathgar, a neighbouring Dublin suburb, to which his mother, Kathleen Synge (*née* Traill), moved following the death of her barrister husband, John Hatch Synge, a man of some independent means. He was reared in a matriarchal society. The house rented by his mother in Orwell Park was next door to his grandmother's home. Mrs Traill was the widow of an evangelical clergyman, Dr Robert Traill, rector of Skull in County Cork, and both she and her daughter were committed to the inflexible religious beliefs held by their ancestors for generations.

The parson grandfather had died in 1847 from an infection contracted from a parishioner with famine fever. The barrister father perished in 1872 from smallpox acquired when visiting a neighbour mildly affected with that disease. Calamities of this kind were common in the nineteenth century and a high infant mortality rate ensured that few families escaped grief. Mrs Synge had lost her eldest son (John William), her elder daughter (Kathleen), and her fourth son (Basil) in infancy. The stock was sound, however, and she herself – though 'dreadfully delicate' when she bore her youngest child[9] – attained the allotted biblical span. Her eldest surviving son, Robert, an engineer who spent some years in Argentina, Edward, an estate agent, Annie (she married Harry Stephens, a solicitor) and Samuel, a medical missionary, lived to be octogenarians. Edmund John Millington (generally called John or Johnnie) was the exception – a sickly child among healthy siblings, an artist (though hardly a bohemian) in a bourgeois family, an unbeliever in a militantly Christian cadre. His mother began to refer to him as 'poor Johnnie' intending the adjective literally, seeing him as deprived of the inestimable riches of the Christian message.

Asthma disrupted his schooling in Upper Leeson Street and Bray. According to his nearest brother, Samuel, the attacks started in Orwell Park when JMS was twelve and continued during their holiday at Dromont in Delgany. 'In after years he used to get it from time to time – a tiring and wearing complaint.'[10] But he had not been permitted to bathe in the sea until July 1881, owing to his delicacy and proneness to coughs and colds, possibly indications of an asthmatic tendency in earlier years.

The practitioners who came to see him, or whom he attended in those years, included a family friend and relative, Dr W.B.B. Scriven of 33 St Stephen's Green, his son, Dr George Scriven, and Dr Henry Oulton of 82 Lower Gardiner Street. His dentist was Mr G.W Yeates of Lower Baggot Street. Later, when the Synges lived in Kingstown (first at 31 Crosthwaite Park and then at Glendalough House, Adelaide Road, Glenageary), he sometimes saw Dr Wright.[11]

The lack of the effective broncho-dilators that nowadays help to relieve asthma must mean that he had to endure many smothering attacks of breathlessness but the compensating feature was that he had more time than other boys of his age to spend in the fresh air, walking and cycling and indulging a growing passion for natural history. He became a bird-watcher, studied insects systematically and in December 1885 joined the newly formed Dublin Naturalists' Field Club.

His wide reading eventually led him to Darwin's *Origin of Species* and to the shattering realization that the highly plausible theory of natural evolution contradicted the account of Genesis and the Garden of Eden on which his mother and grandmother based their conduct of life. He was seized by an agony of doubt – 'the sky seemed to have lost its blue and the grass its green' – and was slow to recover his equanimity.[12]

Adolescence inevitably brought the stresses of post-pubertal development when he was 'absorbed by the ideas that beset men at this period and thought myself a low miscreant because I had a tendency which was really natural and healthy'.[13] He was troubled, too, by creative stirrings that vainly and painfully sought release. 'I wished to be at once Shakespeare, Beethoven and Darwin . . .'.[14]

Synge's real education, according to the poet James Stephens, 'was up in the mountain and out on the bog . . . His professors were the mountainy men and women'[15] of Wicklow, Kerry and Connacht. This was a natural accretion grafted on to the more conventional education obtained when with the help of a tutor he patched together his disrupted schooling and passed the entrance examination to Trinity College. He also enrolled at the Royal Irish Academy of Music, where he was awarded a number of prizes.

He took an undistinguished BA degree in December 1892 and, having already flouted family tradition in the matter of church-going, he earned further disapproval by showing no inclination to follow any profession rewarded by assured remuneration. He refused his brother's offer of a place in the estate agent's office and decided to continue his education in music. Cousin Mary Synge, the only member of the family to speak up for him, arranged that he should stay with the von Eicken sisters, who had a guest-house at Oberwerth, an island in the Rhine, near Koblenz.

For the next ten years he was to spend the winter months on the Continent, returning to Ireland for long family holidays in Wicklow, where every summer Mrs Synge rented a house for the Synges and the Stephenses, who were frequently joined by cousins and friends. Florence Ross, a cousin who lived with the Synges after her mother's death in 1891, was accompanied by her friend and neighbour from 25 Crosthwaite Park, Cherrie

Matheson, when the families were at Castle Kevin in July 1894. Falling deeply in love with Miss Matheson, Synge exalted her as 'the Holy One' and commenced a hesitant courtship.

At this time Samuel Synge was studying medicine at Trinity College and the Adelaide Hospital and was also having lessons in Chinese with the intention of going to China as a missionary. He graduated MB, B.Ch., BAO at the summer examinations in 1895 and became Dr Hayes's resident at Dr Steevens's Hospital in September, also working as *locum tenens* at the National Eye and Ear Infirmary, where he formed a high opinion of Mr (later Sir) Henry Swanzy's ability.

JMS had moved to Würzburg early in 1894 but returned to stay with the von Eickens at Oberwerth in November and in January 1895 took lodgings in Paris, where his spartan existence is reflected in the lines of a poem conceived in 1896:

> There's snow in every street
> Where I go up and down,
> And there's no woman, man or dog
> That knows me in the town.
>
> I know each shop, and all
> These Jews, and Russian Poles,
> For I go walking night and noon
> To spare my sack of coals.[16]

The suggestion that the hardships of this period impaired his health fundamentally cannot be sustained but a faulty diet would have aggravated existing dental decay, imposing limitations which he mentioned wryly to the von Eickens. On the point of 'gnashing' his teeth in a moment of exasperation, 'I remembered in time how bad my teeth were so I only did it in spirit.'[17]

He wrote to Cherrie Matheson in June 1896 proposing marriage and was rejected. They can really have had little in common and as she was a devout member of the Plymouth Brethren his agnosticism was a major obstacle. He remained in her memory as a 'strongly-built man with a rather thick neck and large head, a wonderful face with great luminous sad eyes, and although he was tanned from being constantly out of doors, there was a sort of pallor on his face that gave it a look of delicacy belying his figure, which was that of a hardy mountaineer'.[18]

By now he had forsaken music in favour of languages and literature. He was, indeed, something of a polyglot, speaking German, French and Italian – he visited Rome and Florence in 1896. At Trinity, he had acquired some knowledge of Hebrew and Irish and prior to a visit to Brittany studied Breton. His circle of friends and acquaintances in Paris widened to include Stephen MacKenna, W.B. Yeats, Richard Best and others.

Synge did not attend either his brother's ordination to holy orders in Trinity College chapel or his first sermon at the church in Laragh but Sam was so impressed by some lines written later in an aunt's autograph book that he copied them:

> For mine own soul I would a world create,
> A curious creed, not credulous, divine;
> My soul with lonely loveliness would mate
> Till gleams of glory were to name as mine.[19]

The Rev. Dr Samuel Synge left for China in the autumn of 1896 and took up a post as medical officer to the Church Missionary Hospital, Fuh-Ning, Foochow, South China. He married a Londoner, Dr Mary Harmer, a fellow missionary who took her medical qualifications in Edinburgh. They were to have a daughter and a son.

Since the age of seventeen or so, JMS had enjoyed something of a respite from the headaches, colds and coughs that made him such a sickly child. He was free of asthma for long periods in Kingstown and a course of treatment prescribed by his doctor brother had been helpful. In the latter part of 1897 he noticed that his hair was falling out and that there were swollen lymph glands in his neck. He consulted Dr Wallace Beatty, physician to the Adelaide Hospital, who prescribed a scalp ointment and advised that a surgeon should remove the glands. Mr (later Sir) Charles Ball operated at the nursing-home in Lower Mount Street on 11 December 1897, leaving him free to view the future optimistically. His mother, satisfied to accept that 'he got cold in the glands', was more deeply concerned with his spiritual plight and prayed to God on his behalf: 'Oh I do ask Him to reveal Himself to my dear boy.'[20]

The commonest cause of cervical adenitis (enlarged neck glands) at that period was tuberculosis, but 'TB glands' were painful, matted together and tended to break down and form sinuses, unlike the non-tender, discrete and 'rubbery' glands of the disease named for Thomas Hodgkin (1798–1866) of Guy's Hospital, who described it in 1832.[21] Beatty and Ball (the latter regius professor of surgery at Trinity College) would have been very familiar with the clinical features of Hodgkin's disease and could have confirmed the diagnosis by microscopic examination of a removed gland.[22] The cellular appearance is characteristic.

Hodgkin's disease is progressive if not arrested and at the turn of the century was incurable and fatal, as Beatty and Ball would have known. Their management of Synge's illness was based on a time-honoured medical maxim: *guérir quelquefois, soulager souvent, mais conforter toujours*. Their patient had no dependents, no fortune to dispose of, no major responsibility to burden him. He might remain well for a decade. Why sadden him with the implications of their diagnosis if a euphemism could be substituted?

They may have allowed a senior member of the family, possibly Harry Stephens, part-owner of the nursing-home, to share their secret but Mrs Synge was unaware that her son's future was shadowed when she wrote happily to his brother in China: 'his neck is quite well, quite healed and only a red mark where the cut was, they said they never saw anything heal so quickly'. With motherly concern she kept fires blazing for 'poor Johnnie's' comfort, for he complained that the home climate differed from the warmth at Lower Mount Street, but when she looked at the bills he brought from the nursing-home – 'and the 3 doctors to pay also' – she decided that John would have to pay some of it.[23]

Dr Beatty allowed his patient to return to Paris in mid-January and Synge set out wearing a black wig to cover the temporary baldness following the operation.[24] Later in the year he visited Aran, encouraged to go there by W.B. Yeats, though it may be argued that he would have been attracted there in any case. John Hatch Synge had had property in Galway and the Rev. Alexander Synge, the playwright's uncle, had served as a missionary on Aran and was remembered by the islanders. He stayed for two days at Coole Park with Lady Gregory and his 'A Story from Inishmaan' appeared in the *New Ireland Review* in November 1898.

On his return from his third visit to Aran in October 1900, his mother noticed that although he looked well he had 'one very enlarged gland on his neck just above the collar'.[25] Although anxious about it he does not appear to have sought formal medical advice in Dublin then but did discuss it with Dr James Cree, a Dublin medical graduate who had settled in Paris and had a connection with the Collège des Irlandais. Cree prescribed an ointment but this irritated the swelling and Synge admitted to his mother in April 1901 that he was 'worn and weary and disfigured'.[26] Being sensitive about it he delayed his return to Crosthwaite Park, where his brother Robert and family were staying, until the house was empty. He arrived in Kingstown early in May and visited Dr Parsons, whose ointment and medicine made him feel better. As the swelling now seemed smaller an operation was deferred.[27]

Dr Alfred R. Parsons MD, FRCPI (1865–1952), practised at 27 Lower Fitzwilliam Street. He was assistant physician to Sir Patrick Dun's hospital, moving later to the Royal City of Dublin Hospital, Baggot Street. A colleague has referred to his flair for recognizing uncommon diseases:

Whilst he neglected none of the newer methods of diagnosis he was never led away by any exaggerated or uncritical confidence in their accuracy. He used drugs with skill, but was the first to recognise their limitations, and he was a firm believer in the *vis medicatrix naturae*, and would not overtreat his patients. He was always eager to try new drugs. He did not accept the opinion of others, but tried each one out for himself critically, and formed his own opinion as to whether they were useful or not. Though he had a very large private practice in his heyday, he never aimed at being a fashionable physician, and fame and the amassing of wealth had no attractions for him.[28]

As Synge had asthma in Aran in 1898 and continued to be troubled by episodes of what he conveniently called 'influenza' his mother implored him in vain to give up his '*room* life' in Paris.[29] His first play, *When the Moon Has Set*, was rejected by Lady Gregory but *Riders to the Sea* and *In the Shadow of the Glen*, completed by October 1902, were favourably received. The early part of 1903 was spent in London and he met G.K. Chesterton, John Masefield and other literary figures. He then went on to Paris in order to vacate his little apartment. During the summer of 1903 he was troubled by asthma whenever he visited his mother in County Wicklow, where she rented Tomriland House. Later that year he paid his first visit to County Kerry.

In the Shadow of the Glen was produced at the Molesworth Hall
on 8 October 1903. Padraic Colum recalled that Synge watched
from the back. In response to the cry 'Author! Author!' he walked
forward, mounted the stage and bowed to the audience. His face
was pale, his nervousness evident and there were cheers and hisses.[30]

He was tolerably well until November, when he was suddenly
taken ill with 'influenza and a nasty attack on my lung'.[31] Low-
grade fever prevented his attending the first night of Colum's
Broken Soil. He was recovering slowly when he wrote to Lady
Gregory in mid-December: 'I am getting better now but I cannot
work yet satisfactorily.' He was uncertain as to when he might
complete *The Well of the Saints.*[32]

The first performance of *Riders to the Sea* (25 February 1904)
found him with a toothache caused by a dental abscess which
resulted in a swollen face and kept him in bed for some days, missing the other two performances. The play had a mixed reception
and the family circle echoed the note of general disapproval.
Synge's brother-in-law, Harry Stephens, expressed a preference
for plays like *The Shaughran.*

W.B. Yeats used literary allusions to highlight Synge's struggle:
'What blindness did for Homer, lameness for Hepaestus, asceticism
for any saint you will, bad health did for him by making him ask
no more of life than that it should keep him living, and above all
perhaps by concentrating his imagination upon one thought, health
itself.'[33] But this is to see his handicaps as directives, whereas in
reality, in so far as fortitude permitted, he had tended fatalistically
to ignore the assaults of physical illness. His real achievement was
the triumph over adversity that enabled him to spin his webs of
words, to assemble his splendid imagery despite the obfuscating
forces of fever, lethargy and malaise. 'He spoke with his usual
merry malice about his throat,' Masefield recalled.[34]

The return of well-being brought a renewal of vigour and
optimism which he expressed in a letter to Stephen MacKenna,
who, too, had been ailing:

Don't let yourself talk the bosh that you ain't a strong man no more, we get
waves of good health and bad, but if we aren't organically krank, the bad
waves pass off with a little persuading and leave us live and kicking. I spent last
winter with my ten toes in the grave, and now I'm riding my 70 miles in the
day, with a few mountain ranges thrown in, doing more and doing it more
easily than ever before. Next month maybe I'll be down again.[35]

He worked on *The Well of the Saints*, revising and sharpening the dialogue, and by July 1904 had completed the play. He attended Puck Fair at Killorglin, County Kerry, visited Lady Gregory at Coole Park and postponed a trip to Aran because of smallpox in Kilronan. He came down with 'influenza' in December and was obliged to leave the *pied à terre* he had established in Rathgar and return to the family home in Kingstown.

Meanwhile, Dr and Mrs Samuel Synge had returned to enjoy two years' home leave. They arrived at Kingstown on 7 June 1904. He submitted a thesis, 'Notes on Chinese Medicines',[36] and was awarded the MD by the University of Dublin in December. He took a master's degree in obstetrics (MAO) in the following year.

According to a young nephew whom he scolded for adding sugar to stewed rhubarb, arguing that if sugar were needed God would have put it in the plant, Uncle Sam's 'manner was grave and, though not ill-humoured, he did not suffer frivolity gladly'. He lacked a sense of the ridiculous and when the baby's food was a little sour he ate it for supper so as to observe the admonition 'waste not, want not!'[37]

'I have been so overwhelmed with influenza and rehearsals lately', Synge told D.J. O'Donoghue in January 1905, 'that I have been to see nobody.'[38] *The Well of the Saints* was produced on 4 February by the Abbey players and having established a connection with the *Manchester Guardian* he set off with Jack B. Yeats to report on 'the distress' in the Congested Districts of the West of Ireland. Yeats knew him to be a good companion; he 'was always ready to go anywhere with one and when there to enjoy what came . . .'.[39] From Galway they proceeded to Spiddal where they gave a few halfpence to a poor woman. 'God save you!' she said briefly but when Synge spoke to her in Irish she renewed her thanks. 'That the blessing of God may be on you,' she exclaimed, 'on road and on ridgeway, on sea and on land, on flood and on mountain, in all the kingdoms of the world.'[40]

Synge sent the newspaper three articles a week for four weeks and kept his mother apprised of his health and whereabouts. 'I am all right and have had no Asthma since I left Gorumna on Monday; it is a mysterious complaint. In Gorumna I could have thrown a stone from my bed into the sea, yet I was pretty bad;

and in Carna I was among bogs and I was free from it . . .'.[41] He touched on another aspect of rural Ireland in a letter to Stephen MacKenna: 'There are sides of all that western life the groggy-patriot-publican-general-shop-man who is married to the priest's half sister and is second cousin once-removed of the dispensary doctor, that are horrible and awful.'[42]

Returning to Kingstown in a July heat-wave he was laid up with 'a sort of influenza' but recovered and escaped to Ballyferriter. 'There are very wild Islands – the Blasket Islands – not far from here and I would like to get on them for a while . . . but so far the weather has been so rough I have not even been able to row out to them.' Before long he had arranged to spend a week on the Great Blasket Island.[43]

A further set-back in October was followed by a remission which permitted him to visit his cousin Edward Synge at Byfleet, Surrey, and go on to Cambridge, where the theatre company, on tour, put on all three of his plays in November. Mrs Alfred North Whitehead recalled him as a shabbily clad young man who during luncheon 'said almost nothing and coughed dreadfully'. But when the others moved off to see the College Synge stayed behind with the Whiteheads. 'And then! Three hours he talked brilliantly. We hadn't got his name. But after they were gone, we told each other, "No matter who he is, the man is extraordinary."'[44]

Synge's feelings for Molly Allgood were evident to the whole theatre company by the early months of 1906. The other directors disapproved of the romance and he dared not mention his love of the girl, a nineteen-year-old Catholic without means other than her salary, to his mother. The ensuing frustration was aggravated by Molly's temperament – '*tiff*able' was the euphemism he coined to describe her.

The delayed creative impulses from which his next play was to emerge provided a continuous source of emotional unrest throughout 1905. And that play, the 'notorious' *Playboy of the Western World*, led to the riots, which were followed by a serious exacerbation of the playwright's latent pathology. What can Dr Parsons have thought of this *milieu* so far removed from the ideal?

Bronchitis held him up for ten days in February, as he informed Lady Gregory: 'My lung is not touched however and I have come off well considering.'[45] As the year wore on he was pleased with his progress but planned to take his typewriter with him to County Kerry in order not to interrupt his work. 'I do not think it is worth putting off my holiday . . . as if I do not get a good summer I generally pay for it in the winter in extra bouts of influenza and all its miseries.'[46]

From Glenbeigh, where he had 'a sort of Hay-fever at night' that worried him, he wrote to Molly Allgood almost daily:

My walk yesterday afternoon . . . was wonderful, I was high up on a mountain path looking down a thousand feet of sloping heather into the sea. Then there was Dingle bay perfectly calm and blue, and in the background another line of mountains ending with the Blasquet [*sic*] Islands about 15 miles away. I was up there till sunset and the colour was strangely beautiful. After all while the fine weather lasts it is better to spend my time in places like that than to be fumbling over my play. So far I haven't looked at it . . . [47]

Back in Dublin, his squabbles with Molly so distressed him that he appealed to her: 'Don't you know changeling, that I am an excitable, over-strung fool, – as all writers are, and *have to be*, and don't you love me enough to be a little considerate, and kindly with me even if you do not think that I am always reasonable in what I want you to do? Surely you wouldn't like to worry me into consumption or God knows what?'[48]

Padraic Colum has pointed out that the *Playboy* was written during an active phase of Synge's illness and that it contains 'lines and an incident that reflected the violence of the sick man'.[49]

'My play though in its last agony, is not finished,' he told W.B. Yeats on 4 October, 'and I cannot promise it for any definite day.'[50] The second act proved to be exceptionally difficult but by 18 October he completed it to his satisfaction though at a physical cost, as he explained to Molly: 'I'm not at all well, inside, I'm sorry to say – it is the worry of my play that is knocking me up I think – but I hope I'll be all right tomorrow.'[51]

Towards the end of October, Dr Samuel Synge left for China on the completion of his leave. Presumably he would have spoken to Dr Parsons and have been told all there was to tell about his brother's malady. The latter thought Sam 'one of the best fellows in the world' but so religious that they no longer had much in common. Conscious of his mother's grief at the departure of a favourite son, the playwright stayed close to her until it abated. He

began to have a sense of hopelessness about the *Playboy*. He felt
at his wit's end. 'I must get done with the thing or it will kill
me.'[52] His longing for Molly was a mixture of good and evil
which increased his depression.

Within a matter of days his mood improved. 'I had the best
sleep I have had for weeks [he told Molly] and I feel in great
spirits. The P.Boy is very nearly done I think this week should
get me through with it! Won't that be great?' A reading of the
play was arranged for 13 November. 'Unfortunately I have a
cold and am hoarse and unwell so I won't be able to do myself
justice, I fear.'[53]

The excitement had physical repercussions and after the
reading he had to stay in bed at home. A visit from Molly was
out of the question – propriety forbade that she should enter his
bedroom and downstairs she would face the whole family – 'my
sister and elder brothers and nephews are all in and out. We
would have no peace or satisfaction I'm afraid . . .'.[54] Dr Parsons
was called to see him on the evening of 17 November. He came
at 10.30 p.m. and attributed coughing of blood to a bronchial
disturbance and promised a quick recovery.

'It is all that accursed Playboy,' Synge reflected.[55] He longed
for Molly's letters, which arrived erratically. He wrote to her
frequently. 'I give my letters to you to my mother to send to the
post, and she knew, I think, that I was expecting you yesterday
but we do not speak of you yet. I'm too shaky.' Eventually,
describing her as 'a great friend' of his, he showed Mrs Synge
Molly's photograph. Then screwing up her courage the girl paid
her first visit to Glendalough House on 22 November.[56]

When he called to see Dr Parsons next day he was told to put
off the *Playboy* and go to England for a fortnight. He agreed to
do so and informed Molly accordingly – 'I am not well. The
Playboy is rather a weight on me. I am getting depressed again
now so I had better come to an end.'[57] In England he stayed
with Edward Synge at Byfleet. He felt that the change helped his
work on the *Playboy* but had asthma at night. His cousin's increasing success encouraged him – 'so if I don't kick the bucket I
ought to be able to do good work and plenty of it still'.[58]

He returned to Kingstown on 14 December having 'done very
little to the Playboy' because of asthma.[59] He resumed his work

without delay and continued it daily, including Christmas Day, when he worked until 1.30 p.m and then accompanied his mother to dine at his sister's. 'There were 10 of us in all and we had a pleasant dinner,' he told Molly.[60] Formality and the customs of the close-knit Synge clan evidently precluded her presence at the festivities, such as they were, in Glenageary.

Synge's love for Molly Allgood was highly idealistic, constrained by his innate chivalry and by the mores of his evangelic upbringing; to look at her exalted him but her least departure from his approved code of manners cast him into the depths. Her sore eyes (she attended Mr Henry Swanzy, father of a talented artist, Mary Swanzy) worried him; her dysmenorrhoea (she attended Dr A. Barry) evoked a solicitude bordering on the unhealthy. He urged 'improving' visits to the National Gallery and steered her towards a reading list that would make her distinguished among her peers. He disapproved of her unchaperoned presence in male company and warned her against immoral libertines. 'I know too well how medicals and their like think and speak of the women they run after in Theatres . . .'.[61] Synge's love brought him days of happiness mixed with anguish, and the promise of a delectable consummation.

Miss Allgood's reactions are more difficult to evaluate. What young actress would not have been flattered by the admiration of a rising dramatist who could create parts to set off her talents to perfection? Did the fervour of his emotion distil the heady spirit of love in the alembic of her heart? If so, it must have been cooled from time to time by the lugubrious recital of ailments issuing from the pen of a chronic invalid and by her indifferent reception at Glendalough House. His compliments might bring stars to her eyes, but to be told repeatedly that she had made him broken and 'infinitely wretched' could become something of a bore. Still, she was the central figure in a highly dramatic situation, and that may have had its seductive appeal.

His play went into rehearsal in the New Year and on 7 January Synge mentioned a new complaint – ' My toe is very sore again tonight' – perhaps an attack of gout.[62] 'I have a sort of second edition of influenza,' he told Lady Gregory in the afternoon of 26 January.[63] The *Playboy* had its first production that evening and the Abbey Theatre erupted in a riot. The playwright spent a sleepless night and in the morning felt entitled to borrow the words of Maurya, a character in *Riders to the Sea*: 'It's four fine plays I have though it was a hard birth I had with everyone of them and they coming into the world.' Despite a bad headache he went into Dublin to talk business with Lady Gregory.

He attended the theatre for the next few nights and the *Evening Mail*'s reporter described him as looking 'excited and restless, the perspiration standing out in great beads over his forehead and cheeks'.[64] He defended his play in *The Irish Times*: 'although parts of it are, or are meant to be, extravagant comedy, still a great deal that is in it, and a great deal more that is behind it, is perfectly serious, when looked at in a certain light'.[65]

His cough was worse, leaving him sore all over and as if he had 'ten scarlet devils twisting a crow-bar in the butt of my ribs'.[66] Parsons was called on 4 February and, finding Synge hoarse and wheezing, told him to stay in bed. Dr Parsons came again on 8 February and insisted on further confinement to bed. It may have been during this set-back that Molly dreamed she saw him in a boat . . . She waved to him from the shore, wishing to join him but unable to do so. When she told him, he laughed and said: 'I'm not going to die yet – with the help of God, and I am really not seriously ill.'[67]

Throughout February he remained unwell but towards the end of the month Dr Parsons detected an improvement and favoured activity. Synge mentioned that the players might soon be visiting America, to which the doctor responded by saying it would be just the thing for him. Removal of the glands, followed by a sea voyage, would leave him as strong as a horse. But fever persisted, leading Parsons to examine the sputum for tubercle bacilli, with negative results – much to the patient's relief. 'I'm as happy as the Lord God today . . .', he told Molly, 'and in ten days please Heaven, I shall be trotting you about as usual.'[68]

Regaining his self-confidence, he assured Frank Fay that his troubles were at an end: 'I have been very thoroughly examined by my doctor and there is apparently nothing really the matter with me.[69] His mother had begun to accept that he would marry Molly, though she was still concerned by the prospect of the couple's poverty. He walked outside on 12 March for the first time since the start of this 'complicated influenza' and before long was well enough to complain that the plays of others were being given preference to his.

'I am a little less well today', he informed Molly on 31 March, 'and I am not going out.' Frank Fay's visit had tired him and W.B. Yeats was accepted to call. 'Oh God I wish Yeats wasn't coming today I am so utterly wretched.'[70]

Next day his concern was for Molly. 'I hope you went to Swanzy today you must get your eyes *cured* this time, or you will have endless trouble.' He was agitated, too, by her dysmenorrhoea but added a query by way of postscript: 'I wonder if you make too much of your pains. I don't understand the way you go up and down!'[71] And he himself was advised by Dr Parsons not to take his temperature any more for the present and not to fret if he were a little feverish.

He was startled to learn, as he confided to Stephen MacKenna, that in the West of Ireland the Boards of Guardians were condemning him. 'Irish humour is dead, MacKenna, and I've got influenza.'[72] He had his first bicycle ride for months – 'up through Carrickmines and Kilternan' – on 11 May but Molly left with the players for a five-week tour of England and he fell 'into such a dead abyss of melancholy I got scared'. He worried, too, about the enlarged neck glands, which were unsightly, but Dr Parsons decided to postpone their removal.

Late in May he wrote to Molly from Glendalough House:

It is a wonderful still beautiful evening and I feel as if I ought to write verses but I haven't the energy. There is nearly a half moon, and I have been picturing in my mind how all our nooks and glens and rivers would look, if we were out among them as we should be! Do you ever think of them? Ever think of them I mean not as places that you've been to, but as places that are there still, with the little moon shining, and the rivers running, and the thrushes singing, while you and I, God help us, are far away from them. I used to sit over my sparks of fire in Paris picturing glen after glen in my mind, and river after river – there are rivers like the Annamoe that I fished in till I knew every stone and eddy – and then one goes on to see a time when the rivers will be there and the thrushes, and we'll be dead surely.[73]

When he learned that, against his wishes, she had shared 'digs' with the men in Glasgow he felt sick with anguish, and quite broken and dejected. His emotional distress was aggravated by a painful knee but when this improved he went to stay with Jack B. Yeats in Devonshire, enjoying the landscapes in Wicklow and

Wexford on the train journey to Rosslare after the rain had
stopped: 'My spirits are going UP. The country is wonderful,
masses of bluebells, and wet green trees and ferns everywhere.
It's wonderful after the long imprisonment I've had.'[74]

From Strete in Devon he moved to London and was shown
around the House of Commons by Stephen Gwynn MP. The
June weather was hot and oppressive. He slept poorly and felt ill.
Back in Dublin he consulted Dr Parsons, who examined his lungs
and found nothing amiss. 'He thinks however that I ought to get
the glands out and recover myself a bit before I get married.'[75]

Mrs Synge thought it would be improper for him to share a
holiday cottage in Glencree with his fiancée and her sister but
when he spoke to her about Molly's intimate problems she was
reassuring in a motherly way. 'She seems to have known a lot of
cases like yours, Mrs X, Mrs Z and Miss Y and so on and they all
got well and lived happily ever afterwards.'[76] That morsel of confidence between the mother and the playwright son with whom
she had so few common bonds was treasured by Mrs Synge and
relayed privily to Dr Samuel Synge in China.

Determined to get rid of the cough that had racked him for
five months, and longing to get away from the Irish weather, he
thought of spending August abroad. The doctor had advised a
dry bracing place. 'Have play ideas at the back of my mind [he
told Lady Gregory] but I'm not doing anything yet, as I want to
get well first.'[77] His mood varied with the weather. Cycling over
the Wicklow hills on 23 July he encountered soaking rain but
after a few warm days he felt in better health than at any time
since his trip to Kerry in the previous summer. Asthma then
recurred and kept him awake.

His plans for a cycling tour of Brittany with Henri Lebeau, a
French university teacher, fell through on account of further
respiratory attacks and he spent many lonely, wretched days on
his own in Glendalough House. 'I think I'm better today [he
told Molly] but I'm not sure. I'm going out for a while I can't
stand another lonely day in here. I thought yesterday would
never end, – sitting in these empty rooms from 9 in the morning
till 11 at night.'[78]

Synge's physical appearance has been variously outlined and
there are many vignettes smudged or otherwise to choose from;

where Bernard Shaw's instant glance saw 'a face like a blacking-brush', John Masefield looked more closely: 'It was a grave dark face with a good deal in it . . . The mouth, not well seen below the moustache, had a great play of humour in it.' George Moore recalled him

sitting thick and straight in my armchair, his large uncouth head, and flat, ashen-coloured face with two brown eyes looking at me not unsympathetically. A thick stubbly growth starts out of a strip of forehead like black twigs out of the head of a broom. I see a ragged moustache and he sits bolt upright in my chair, his legs crossed, his great country shoes spreading over my carpet.

John Butler Yeats, kinder and wiser than Moore, looked more deeply at the subject he painted in his St Stephen's Green studio:

He was a well-built, muscular man, with broad shoulders, carrying his head finely. He had large, light-hazel eyes which looked straight at you. His conversation . . . had the charm of absolute sincerity . . . He neither deceived himself nor anybody else, and yet he had the enthusiasm of a poet.[79]

'There was nothing about Synge to make a crowd throw up a hat,' Padraic Colum said. He had called on him at Crosthwaite Park ('a lifeless square'), coming to know him better when he moved to Rathmines to be closer to the theatre. They sometimes walked together in the afternoons. 'He had a laugh that was half grim, half good-humoured.'[80]

Oliver St John Gogarty, a joyous and irreverent man, found Synge 'inscrutable' and lacking robustness. They happened to meet in the street in August 1907 – 'he says I ought to get the glands out as soon as ever I can', Synge reported to Molly, 'and that I will be all right then.'[81]

Parsons and Ball agreed that surgery was now indicated, suppressing their fears that it was too late to be beneficial. The enlarged lymph glands that formed such an ugly lump in the neck were possibly only 'the tip of the ice-berg', if that gross metaphor is suitable to describe the malign and subtle process that had invaded Synge's tissues, spreading, perhaps, through chains of glands into the centre of the chest, transforming those homogeneous structures into grey or pink masses resembling fish-flesh.

The diseased glands if viewed by an inexpert microscopist might appear as baffling as an abstract painting until the pleomorphic cellular infiltration was pointed to by a pathologist and explained as a disorderly assembly of cells, varied in size and shape, replacing the normal, stolid lymphocytes; an apparently purposeless usurpation by large cells with blistered nuclei, by pink eosinophils, by mononuclear cells with indented nuclei and by giant cells equipped with many large nuclei (the 'Dorothy Reed cells' described in 1902); a sinister, morbid extravaganza to delight some Des Esseintes of the laboratory for whom a plasma cell is no less beautiful than a topaz, who sees disease and distress objectively as the tax exacted by nature for the infinite wonders inherent in protoplasm, a dreadful excrescence governed by its own laws and periodicities.

The operation was done at the nursing-home in Lower Mount Street, now called the 'Elpis', and the patient wrote to his fiancée on 20 September: 'I'm getting on very well but it's terribly slow. I'm afraid of having people in to see me JUST YET as I'm a bit too weak still . . . Sir C. Ball is going to take off the dressings tomorrow and then if all is well perhaps he'll let me up.'[82]

He convalesced at Ventry, County Kerry, but could ill afford the trip because Mrs Synge made no contribution to the nursing-home expenses and the holiday was spoiled to some extent by asthma. 'Certainly I am an afflicted poor devil. I am all right now however fortunately it only takes me at night.'[83]

On his return to Glendalough House a surge of creativity enabled him 'in great spirits and joy' to write ten pages of a new play based on the legend of Deirdre and the sons of Usna. He kept Molly informed of his progress with what he planned to be a three-act drama:

I haven't had dinner today yet; but I've been working at Deirdre till my head is going round. I was too taken up with her yesterday to write to you – I got her into such a mess I think I'd have put her in the fire only that I want to write a part for YOU, so you mustn't be jealous of her.[84]

Within a week he completed the second rough draft of the play and fine weather allowed him to get out on his bicycle. 'I had a long ride this afternoon – the country was radiantly bright and wonderful and I was as happy as seven kings. I had nearly forgotten what it was like to be in good health, and to have hearty spirits.'[85]

This reassertion of well-being was tempered by fundamental difficulties – 'I am working myself sick with Deirdre or whatever you call it. It is a very anxious job. I don't want to make a failure' – those related to his play and others arising from the unconsummated love affair: 'I cannot live this way any longer – I nearly died of loneliness and misery last night while you ought to be here to comfort me and cheer me up.'[86]

He walked to Loughlinstown on 23 November, returning by train from Killiney 'in time for a bout at Deirdre'. He wrote seven pages on 26 November but was bored by his mother's visitor at Glendalough House, a lady missionary, and the effort of making small talk at meals. He had room for only one thing in his mind.

I am squirming and thrilling and quivering with the excitement of writing Deirdre and I *daren't* break the thread of composition by going out to look for digs and moving into them at this moment . . . One thing is absolutely certain as soon as ever we find a digs now we must be married *even if you have no holidays*. Let me get Deirdre out of danger – she may be safe in a week – then Marriage in God's Name. Would you mind a *registry office* if that saves time? I don't know whether it does or not . . . I went to the dentist yesterday, but there was nothing serious to be done.[87]

The storm of creativity kept the playwright buoyant, unconcerned by a slight recurrence of the swelling in the neck. When consulted on 2 December, Dr Parsons pronounced him to be *grand*.[88] There was nothing to account for a new symptom – 'some curmurring in his guts', Synge called it later, borrowing from Robert Burns[89] – but this was actually the initial manifestation of the presence of Hodgkin's disease in the abdominal organs.

'Deirdre is getting on I think, but slowly [he told Molly on 10 December]. I over-worked myself for a while and I'm taking it easier now. In any case at this stage one cannot go fast.'[90] He took an active part in the theatre management, unaware of Lady Gregory's note to Yeats: 'We shall have to snub Synge and Molly in the end – her being late in assignations with him is no excuse for her upsetting rehearsals.'[91]

As 1908 opened he continued to work obsessively on his play. 'I am working at D again – I can't keep away from her, till I get her right . . . '. He was in good spirits and satisfied with what he had written but told Holbrook Jackson that it was still 'too vague to be put into paragraphs'.[92] When Frank and Willie Fay resigned on 13 January 1908 he took rooms at 47 York Road, Upper Rathmines, to be closer to the theatre. 'Poor Yeats with his bad sight

and everything is very helpless, and I have to look after him a bit' –
but he admired the senior poet's flair for bossing the carpenters.[93]

'I am glad to say that I am in very good health this year', he
told a correspondent, 'and nearly through another play.' But his
innards continued to trouble him and, having eaten fruit to no
avail, he felt an operation would be required. 'I told him I could
not pay for another and I did not think it was necessary,' Mrs
Synge confided to her eldest son, Robert, who had returned to
live in Ireland.[94]

Now it was her turn to consult a doctor, having noticed a
lump in the groin in February 1908. Dr Beatty told her a white
lie, saying it was a hernia, a well-intentioned deception repeated
by his surgical colleague. But when Mr Gordon[95] did the biopsy
at the Elpis Nursing-Home the diagnosis they must have suspected
was confirmed – Mrs Synge had cancer. She accepted a less stark
explanation and contentedly planned a summer of recovery at
Tomriland House. She discussed the question of John's marriage
with him, having decided to come to terms with the inevitable.[96]

He proposed to call the play *Deirdre of the Sorrows*. He expected
to have it ready for production by autumn but in April Dr Parsons
found a lump in his side and began to talk of an investigation to
clarify its significance. His mother was shocked by the change in
his appearance – 'he is thin and white, a pallor I do not like to
see'[97] – and Sir Charles Ball agreed to operate in the Elpis
Nursing-Home on 5 May.

'Sir Charles Ball would not say what he thought my trouble
was [Synge told Lady Gregory], but he looked glum enough
over me this morning. They do not really know of course what
they may find when they go to work.'[98]

In the absence of modern methods of endoscopy, imaging and
needle biopsy, the 'laporotomy' or exploratory operation was
formerly an accepted and useful diagnostic expedient but in view
of what was already known in Synge's case the surgeon cannot
have been surprised to encounter an inoperable tumour. Dr Parsons
broke the news to Mrs Synge and for some days the patient's life
was actually in immediate danger.

Synge's post-operative course was stormy, as his mother
explained to Robert: 'Things did not go right after the operation
and until last Sunday Sir Charles Ball had no hope of our dear

boy's life . . . On Sunday morning, Dr Ball took out the stitches, and immediately the wound opened and a great discharge came from it, and that saved his life.' This transformed the situation, to everyone's relief. 'God has permitted it all to happen,' Mrs Synge told Robert, 'so I can say nothing . . . '.[99]

Dr Parsons explained to Mrs Synge that the tumour was adherent – 'it would not have been desirable to have attempted its removal'.[100] An obstruction had been corrected by enterostomy but the prognosis was hopeless and deterioration must be expected. This need not be revealed to the patient and Synge was actually led to believe that the tumour had been removed, necessitating a large incision and cutting the bowel.

Was this justifiable? Parsons and Ball certainly believed it to be and their 'deception' preserved Synge's creativity. Today, with cures and remedies tumbling from the cornucopia, complete candour must obtain between doctor and patient while for terminal situations the ministrations of counsellors are beneficial.

He was slow to regain his strength and healing of the wound was delayed. He remained in the nursing-home until 6 July, when, as Mrs Synge was away and in declining health, he went to stay with his sister at Silchester House around the corner from Glendalough House. Ever frugal, he went out to Sandycove by tram and took a cab to Silchester Road. A night of fever alarmed Mrs Stephens, who contacted Sir Charles Ball – 'he came down to see me in his motor. He couldn't find anything wrong . . . '.[101]

Synge pottered in the garden, walked a little in the neighbourhood and went to Bray on 21 July, but he was alarmed and annoyed by a variety of aches and pains. He had learned how to dress the wound but felt unskilled in this procedure. On 23 July he went to see the surgeon and reported the visit to Molly: 'I'm not very well with all Ball's talk and I had a worse night than ever last night. I think I'll go to see Parsons on Monday.'[102]

He found the wound closed one day, open the next. As Parsons and Ball both were away he consulted the latter's son, Mr C.A.K Ball.[103] 'He found, he thinks, the cause of the discharge – an *un*important one if he is right but he does not really know what my severe pains are from. I liked him very much and I am to go back to him in a few days if I am not better. He takes more trouble and is much gentler than the old man.'[104]

A visit from W.B. Yeats had made him feel 'like getting back into the current of life again' but his letter to Stephen MacKenna on 12 August was disconsolate:

> I've been pining for the sight of your face all these weeks, but somehow from the uncertainty of my insides I've never had the decision necessary to say 'tomorrow I'll have MacKenna,' and then to write to you to fix a time. In fact I've not been very well and I've been sitting quaking in the garden like a sear and yellow leaf. The doctors say I'm a very interesting case and generally patronise my belly – to think that I used once to write 'Playboys,' MacKenna, and now I'm a bunch of interesting bowels!
>
> My mother has come home unwell from the country so I return to Glendalough House tomorrow.[105]

He resumed work on 'Deirdre' towards the end of the month. By early October the doctors' bills had arrived – Parsons £20, Elpis £37, Ball £57 – and proved difficult for him to meet with his slender means. A poem evoked by Molly's reply to his question 'Will you go to my funeral?', posed by way of a macabre joke, was judged to be magnificent by W.B. Yeats:

> I asked if I got sick and died, would you
> With my black funeral go walking too,
> If you'd stand close to hear them talk or pray
> While I'm let down in that steep bank of clay.
> And, No, you said, for if you saw a crew
> Of living idiots, pressing round that new
> Oak coffin – they alive, I dead beneath
> That board, – you'd rave and rend them with your teeth.[106]

Parsons forbade him to go by sea to the Mediterranean in case *mal de mer* would wreak havoc with internal structures. He set off instead to stay with the von Eickens at Oberwerth. 'I am only beginning to realize what a wreck this business has left me [he wrote to Molly]. However I won't be downcast – '.[107] At Oberwerth he walked in the woods, resting at every seat to ease his 'poor ripped belly and all the time seeking inspiration for Deirdre'.

On his return from a walk on 26 October he was given Robert Synge's telegram: 'Mother has passed away funeral Thursday don't come unless strong enough for journey.' He remained in Germany until 5 November and, arriving in Kingstown two days later, felt inexpressibly sad in empty Glendalough House. His sister explained his material benefit. His share of the property was worth £1500, which, when added to what he had already, would give him an annual income of £110.

Self-preservation is among man's deepest instincts. Hope is not easily surrendered and even those who have reached a stage of extreme debility and cachexia can cling to ardent expectations astonishing to healthy onlookers. Synge's amazing courage enabled him to trust in the future. Almost to the end he held on to hope, riding meanwhile a see-saw of optimism and despair. Some weeks after his mother's death a sardonic angel was at his elbow when he wrote the following lines:

> I read about the Blaskets and Dunquin,
> The Wicklow towns and fair days I've been in.
> I read of Galway, Mayo, Aranmore,
> And men with kelp along a wintry shore.
> Then I remembered that that 'I' was I,
> And I'd a filthy job – to waste and die.[108]

No more accurate prognosis could have been offered than 'to waste and die', but soon Synge shrugged off this mood of abject dejection. He compiled notes for changes in 'Deirdre' and was pleased with the scene between Deirdre and Lavarcham at the beginning of Act II. He visited Parsons on 4 December. The doctor may have curbed his expectations by insisting that recovery would be slow. 'They say it will be a year or near it [Synge told T.P. Gill] before I am quite comfortable.'[109]

'I've done the usual amount of Deirdre and had the usual belly-aches and taken my usual little walks, bad cess to the lot of them.'[110] Synge's interminable recital of woe appears to have irritated and upset Molly Allgood, who may not have always succeeded in dissembling or in appreciating the heroic struggle he had made in getting so far with his new play:

I feel humiliated [he wrote to her on Christmas Eve] that I showed you so much of my weakness and emotion yesterday. I will not trouble you any more with complaints about my health – you have taught me that I should not – but I think I owe it to myself to let you know that if I am so 'selfpitiful' I have some reason to be so as Dr Parsons' report of my health, though uncertain, was much more unsatisfactory than I thought it well to tell you. I only tell you now because I am unable to bear the thought that you should think of me with the contempt I saw in your face yesterday.[111]

When he wrote to Lady Gregory on 3 January 1909, he reported good progress with 'Deirdre'. 'I only work a little every day as

I suffer more than I like with indigestion and general uneasiness inside – I hope it is only because I haven't quite got over the shock of the operation – the doctors are vague and don't say much that is definite.'[112]

Seumas O'Sullivan, the poet, was amazed to encounter Synge looking at bookshops on the quays on 5 January, having learned that he was ill. He had come into the city to see Dr Parsons, who was called away. When Parsons saw him next day he encouraged him to cycle, prescribed a tonic and told him to see Ball. The latter resorted to an old-fashioned remedy, castor-oil.

Sir C.B. was evidently right in what he thought – or part of it – but I'm not cured yet, so I'll have to give myself more doses, God help me. However if that will set me right then may Heaven's eternal fragrance fall on Castor Oil. I wonder if you can follow all this. I've been thinking about you a great deal with your little socks for me, and all your little attentions and I'm ready to go down on my knees to your shadow – if I met it in a dry place, – I think I'm drunk with Castor oil![113]

Padraic Colum's last meeting with Synge was a chance encounter in the street. He walked with him to Westland Row railway station, where Synge was to take a train to Glenageary. Colum noticed the sunken face and the intensity with which he spoke of the play he was writing, having reached the third act. 'He began to tell me about this act: there would be an open grave on the stage.' Colum demurred but Synge explained that he had been close to death 'and that the grave was a reality to him, and it was the reality in the tragedy he was writing'. Colum still thought it inappropriate – especially now that he said he was getting well.[114]

As it was now obvious to Robert Synge that his brother was dreadfully ill, he made him write to Dr Parsons and arrange for the physician to call to Glendalough House. As there was no improvement towards the weekend, Parsons decided that he should return to the Elpis Nursing-Home and he did so on 2 February. 'They say I'm getting on well', he told Lolly Yeats two weeks later, 'but I'm in bed still.'[115]

Molly came to see him daily and there were other visitors. He read the Bible but refused to see a clergyman and when the matron sent a minister along they discussed the weather. He was determined to remain earthbound. 'Not being sure of heaven', he said, 'I'll stay here as long as I can.' A few days before his death he was moved to a sunny room with a distant view of the Dublin Mountains. He would probably have been too fatigued and languid then to recall an impulse that had prompted him at a moment of danger in a storm-tossed curragh almost to welcome the prospect of a sudden death: 'What a difference to die here with the fresh sea saltness in my hair than to struggle in soiled sheets with a smell of my own illness in my nostril . . .'.[116] A death like Shelley's instead of Heine's long-drawn agony on his 'mattress-grave' in Paris.

His favourite nurse, a Catholic, made him say prayers night and morning. He called her his 'tidy nurse' and sang her praises to Dr Parsons. He was still conscious when she sprinkled him with holy water. He asked was she baptizing him and added, 'Perhaps it is best so.' He is said to have murmured, towards the end, 'God have mercy on me. God forgive me.'

According to the dramatic account of Synge's last moments given by W.B. Yeats, he spoke to the nurse in the early morning of 24 March: '"It's no use fighting death any longer," he said and turned on his side and died.' It is far more likely that no words were spoken but that the night-nurse watching her unconscious patient through the small hours noticed a change in his breathing and listened to it weaken until the arrival of a moment when she could not say whether he was alive or dead.

John Millington Synge was buried in Mount Jerome Cemetery, the sombrely suited, bowler-hatted relatives standing apart from the small group of writers and theatre people who came to say adieu. The immediate business of Synge's life was then not quite ended, for on 13 January 1910 *Deirdre of the Sorrows* was produced at the Abbey Theatre with Molly playing Deirdre. The audience included young Walter Starkie, who a few years earlier attended the *Playboy*'s first night and saw the author as 'a forlorn figure in the midst of pandemonium'.[117]

Deirdre's first night remained a potent memory for Starkie, who recalled the poignant acting of Molly Allgood.[118] He had discerned 'a ghostly quality, as though the slight brown-eyed girl with her pale face, the embodiment of tragedy, still lingered under the hypnotic spell of the dead author . . .'.[119] Her voice was redolent of pathos when she said, 'I have put away sorrow like a shoe that is worn out and muddy, for it is I have had a life that will be envied by great companies.'[120]

NOTES

1. John Millington Synge, *Collected Works* (ed. Alan Price), vol. II (London 1966), p. 23.
2. *Ibid.*, p. 39.
3. *Ibid.*, p. 40.
4. *Ibid.*, p. 42.
5. *Ibid.*, p. 43.
6. *Ibid.*, p. 43.
7. TCD MS. 4382 ff 2–5.
8. *Collected Works*, II, p. 4.
9. Edward Stephens, *My Uncle John* (ed. Andrew Carpenter) (London 1974), p. 42.
10. Samuel Synge, *Letters to My Daughter* (Dublin 1932), p. 56.
11. When old Mrs Traill died early in 1890 Mr and Mrs Harry Stephens, who had lived with her in a house adjoining that occupied by the Synges (and united to it by a door in the party wall), moved to 29 Crosthwaite Park, Kingstown (now Dún Laoghaire). The Synges joined the Stephens at 31 Crosthwaite Park in January 1891, having moved temporarily in October 1890 to 9 Crosthwaite Park.

    Harry Stephens, a prosperous solicitor, resided at opulent Silchester House, Glenageary, from 1906, and, to remain close to her daughter and grandchildren, Mrs Synge moved to nearby Glendalough House in Adelaide Road, Glenageary, on 19 July 1906.

    JMS made two attempts to set up independently: on 6 February 1906 he lodged at 57 Rathgar Road; on 2 February 1908 he took rooms at 47 York Road, Rathmines.
12. *Collected Works*, II, p. 10.
13. *Ibid.*, p. 12. For further expressions of the psychological trauma of puberty see James Joyce, *A Portrait of the Artist as a Young Man*, where Stephen Dedalus asks: 'Who made it to be like that, a bestial part of the body able to understand bestially and desire bestially?'; and W.B. Yeats's description of how sexual arousal 'filled me with loathing of myself' (*Memoirs*, ed. Denis Donoghue, 1972, p. 72).
14. *Ibid.*, p. 14.
15. E.H. Mikhail (ed.), *J. M. Synge, Interviews and Recollections* (London 1983), p. 9.
16. *Collected Works*, I, p. 63.
17. Ann Saddlemyer (ed.), *The Collected Letters of John Synge*, vol. I (Oxford 1983), p. 9.
18. Mikhail, *op. cit.*, p. 3.
19. Samuel Synge, *op. cit.*, p. 99.

20. Stephens, *op. cit.*, p. 109.
21. Ellenborough King, age ten, was one of two cases described by Thomas Hodgkin in his classic paper, 'On Some Morbid Appearances of the Absorbent Glands and Spleen' (*Medical and Chirurgical Transactions*, London [1832], 17: 68). 'The glands on the left side of the neck were swollen, as well as those on the right . . .'.

    Curator of the museum and lecturer in pathology at Guy's Hospital, Hodgkin was a member of the Society of Friends and followed their customs in speech and dress.
22. Sir Charles Bent Ball, Bart (1851–1916), surgeon to Sir Patrick Dun's Hospital and regius professor of surgery in the University of Dublin, was the author of *The Rectum and Anus, Their Diseases and Treatment* (1894) and *The Rectum, Its Diseases and Developmental Defects* (1908). Sir Robert Ball FRS, the astronomer, was his elder brother.

    Wallace Beatty (1853–1923) served the Adelaide Hospital for more than forty years as physician and dermatologist, confining himself to the latter speciality after middle age because of increasing deafness. He was honorary professor of dermatology at the University of Dublin and author of *Lectures on Diseases of the Skin* (1922).

    Beatty was born at Halifax, Nova Scotia, the son of a railway engineer who died in 1857 as the result of an accident in the Crimea. He was educated at Dungannon School and TCD.
23. Samuel Synge, *op. cit.*, pp. 152–3.
24. Stephens, *op. cit.*, p. 114.
25. *Ibid.*, p. 134.
26. *Letters*, I, p. 44.
27. Stephens, *op. cit.*, p. 143.
28. Parsons's obituarist (*Irish Journal of Medical Science* [1952], 138–9) was the playwright's nephew, Professor Victor Millington Synge MD, FRCPI, physician to the Royal City of Dublin Hospital. Having praised his colleague and outlined his career he asks:

    And what of Parsons the man? . . . He was a spartan in body who denied himself the seductive stimulation of tobacco and alcohol and who, old as he was, took his cold bath every day in the bitterest winter – truly a Spartan in his inflexible will power, but an Athenian in his broad cultural outlook and genius of mind.

29. *Letters*, I, p. 43.
30. Mikhail, *op. cit.*, p. 64.
31. *Letters*, I, p. 70.
32. *Ibid.*, p. 71.
33. Mikhail, *op. cit.*, p. 57.
34. *Ibid.*, p. 83.
35. *Letters*, I, p. 87.
36. Samuel Synge, 'Notes on Chinese Medicines', *Dublin Journal of Medical Science* (1904), 119: 184–9.
37. Stephens, *op. cit.*, p. 168.
38. *Letters*, I, p. 104.

39. *Collected Works*, III, p. 402.
40. *Ibid.*, II, p. 287.
41. *Letters*, I, p. 114.
42. *Ibid.*, p. 116.
43. *Ibid.*, p. 119.
44. *Ibid.*, p. 103.
45. *Ibid.*, p. 159.
46. *Ibid.*, p. 185.
47. *Ibid.*, p. 198.
48. *Ibid.*, p. 207.
49. Mikhail, *op. cit.*, p. 68.
50. *Letters*, I, p. 211.
51. *Ibid.*, p. 220.
52. *Ibid.*, p. 225.
53. *Ibid.*, p. 234.
54. *Ibid.*, p. 235.
55. *Ibid.*, p. 136.
56. *Ibid.*, p. 239.
57. *Ibid.*, p. 244.
58. *Ibid.*, p. 251.
59. *Ibid.*, p. 262.
60. *Ibid.*, p. 267.
61. *Ibid.*, p. 249.
62. *Ibid.*, p. 280.
63. *Ibid.*, p. 284.
64. Mikhail, *op. cit.*, p. 39.
65. *Letters*, I, p. 268.
66. *Ibid.*, p. 290.
67. *Ibid.*, p. 290.
68. *Ibid.*, p. 307.
69. *Ibid.*, p. 308.
70. *Ibid.*, p. 324.
71. *Ibid.*, p. 325.
72. *Ibid.*, p. 330.
73. *Ibid.*, p. 353.
74. *Ibid.*, p. 364.
75. *Ibid.*, p. 368.
76. *Ibid.*, p. 371.
77. *Letters*, II, p. 7.
78. *Ibid.*, p. 31.
79. Mikhail, *op. cit.*, *passim*.
80. *Ibid.*, p. 63.
81. *Ibid.*, II, p. 33.
82. *Ibid.*, p. 59.
83. *Ibid.*, p. 68.
84. *Ibid.*, p. 75.

85. *Ibid.*, p. 76.
86. *Ibid.*, p. 79.
87. *Ibid.*, p. 92.
88. According to Victor Millington Synge, his senior colleague, Dr Parsons,

    never believed in telling his patients much about their ailments and few dared to question him. He was beloved by them all, from the wheezy septuagenarian whom he was too kind-hearted to discharge from the hospital in the cold winter months, to the small children in the nursery who greeted him every morning with shouts of joy.

    Parson was an octogenarian when the present writer attended his class at Baggot Street Hospital; he was a most inspiring teacher. Another pupil, Dr E. MacCarthy, sent her valedictory lines to the *Irish Journal of Medical Science* (1952), 139:

    > His was the green old age of the god
    > that sadly watched a world decay.
    > Now the dark ferry paddles him away,
    > but as black Charon dips his blade
    > the god will say:
    > 'He is the immortal
    > *I* the shade.'

89. *Letters*, II, p. 227.
90. *Ibid.*, p. 101.
91. *Ibid.*, p. 112.
92. *Ibid.*, p. 139.
93. *Ibid.*, p. 135.
94. *Ibid.*, p. 145.
95. Thomas E. Gordon FRCSI was elected surgeon to the Adelaide Hospital in 1896, promoted from the assistant surgeoncy he held since 1892. He was appointed to the chair of surgery in Dublin University in 1916. He retired from the Adelaide Hospital in 1929 and died shortly afterwards.
96. Stephens, *op. cit.*, p. 200.
97. *Letters*, II, p. 153.
98. *Ibid.*, p. 154.
99. Stephens, *op. cit.*, p. 202.
100. *Letters*, II, p. 156.
101. *Ibid.*, p. 162.
102. *Ibid.*, p. 171.
103. Mr Charles Arthur Kinahan Ball FRCSI (1877–1945) was then assistant surgeon to Dun's Hospital. He succeeded to his father's title in 1916 and became regius professor of surgery in 1933. His marriage to Elizabeth Wilson of Berkeley, California, was childless and the title passed to his brother, Nigel, a former professor of botany at the University of Colombo.
104. *Letters*, II, p. 180.
105. *Ibid.*, p. 182.
106. *Collected Works*, I, p. 64.
107. *Letters*, II, p. 232.
108. *Collected Works*, I, p. 66.
109. *Letters*, II, p. 232.

110. *Ibid.*, p. 235.
111. *Ibid.*, p. 236.
112. *Ibid.*, p. 242.
113. *Ibid.*, p. 249.
114. Mikhail, *op. cit.*, p. 68.
115. *Letters*, II, p. 253.
116. Stephens, *op. cit.*, p. 122.
117. Mikhail, *op. cit.*, p. 132.
118. In 1911 Molly Allgood married G. H. Mair, who worked with the *Manchester Guardian*. They had two children, John and Pegeen. After Mair's death she married an actor, Francis McDonnell, toured America and worked on the stage and in films and radio in London.
119. Mikhail, *op. cit.*, p. 132.
120. John Millington Synge, *The Complete Plays* (ed. T.R. Henn) (London 1981), p. 275.

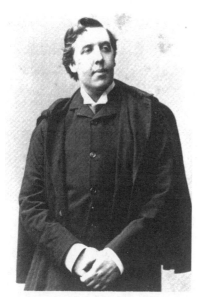

7. Oscar Wilde *c.* 1891 (Courtesy of the William Andrews
   Clark Library)

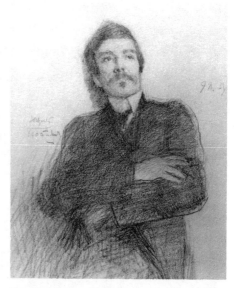

8. John Millington Synge by John Butler Yeats (Courtesy of
   the National Gallery of Ireland)

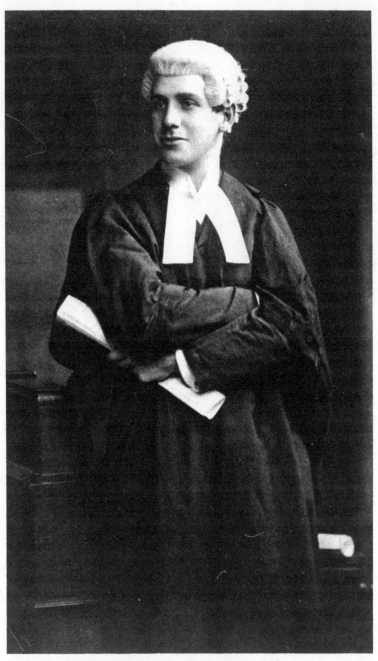

9. T.M. Kettle BA, BL (Photo by Lafayette)

*Tom Kettle, 1880–1916**

A plaque on 25 Northumberland Road, Dublin, records the death there of Lieutenant Michael Malone at Easter 1916. The adjoining house is free of nationalistic adornments but should Dublin Corporation show an interest in the see-saw of Irish sacrifices it could attach a notice: formerly the residence of Lieutenant Thomas Michael Kettle, killed at the Battle of the Somme in 1916. This would provide an interesting confrontation of two traditions in Irish history. The importance of Kettle's career is the failure of his undeviating constitutionalism and personal sacrifice to move his political opponents, which goes some way to explain the inevitability of the insurrection.

EARLY YEARS

Tom Kettle, the third son of Andrew Kettle, one of the founders of the Land League, and his wife, Margaret McCourt, was born on 9 February 1880. His birthplace is usually given as Artane but in his father's memoirs, *Material for Victory*, it is stated that most of the family were born in Millview, Malahide. Andrew Kettle, who was himself born at Drynan House, Swords, in 1833, farmed at Drynan and later at Kilmore, Artane; Millview, Malahide; and Newtown, St Margaret's.[1]

I have recovered no traces of Tom Kettle's infancy or early childhood and my first picture of him comes from the pages of Oliver St John Gogarty, who described Kettle's daily arrival at the O'Connell School, North Richmond Street, in a governess cart:

* Presented to the Old Dublin Society, 21 March 1990, and published in the *Dublin Historical Record* (1990), 43, 85–98.

Tom Kettle was dark. He had eyes like the eyes of Robbie Burns, the eyes of genius. He wore dark gray clothes with three buttons on the sides of his knee britches such as all schoolboys wore. He would not hail any of the other boys when he came to the school, although his eyes looked here and there. It was as if he already had things in his mind that were beyond the school. He moved about in his governess cart, not to gather his books but because his energy made him restless . . . [2]

Tom's eldest brother, Andy, followed the farming tradition. Larry, the next boy, who was to become Dublin's Electrical Engineer, was, like Tom, a prizewinner at O'Connell's and also at Clongowes, where they moved to in 1894. In the Intermediate Education Board's junior grade examination that summer, Tom was awarded the maximum marks in both algebra and Euclid.

At Clongowes Tom developed a liking for cricket which was to get him into hot water later with enthusiasts for Gaelic games, but his favourite sport was cycling. The school's debating society was the forum in which he learned how to speak in public and his first publication, an essay on Owen Roe O'Neill, appeared in *The Clongownian*.[3]

He continued to excel in the classroom, taking the Intermediate Board's prize for English composition in the senior grade in 1897, his last year at school, in which year the middle grade prize went to James Joyce, then in Belvedere. Kettle also won a gold medal for first place in the senior grade, a gold medal for English and second place in French and entered the university with a formidable academic reputation.

University College, St Stephen's Green, then under the direction of the Jesuit order, prepared students for the degrees of the Royal University. The institution was impecunious and poorly appointed, lacking a library but managing to compensate for its material deficiencies and boasting a higher success rate than its rival, the Queen's Colleges in Belfast, Cork and Galway. Many of its alumni achieved high positions in Irish public life.

By the time he arrived there, Tom Kettle possessed an abundance of attractive qualities. 'He spoke to you', Gogarty said, 'as from some Elysium, where everyone was merry, unmalicious, and full of gay wisdom.'[4] He had friendly brown eyes and an eager smile in which there was a good deal of raillery – 'raillery of himself as well as of others' – Padraic Colum recalled.[5] He was tall, well-built and handsome; his complexion was sallow, his hair sleek and black, his mouth wide and mobile, his forehead large and well-moulded.

Kettle's teachers warmed to him. He was especially influenced by Father Tom Finlay, economist and editor of the *New Ireland Review*. The revival of the Literary and Historical Society – the celebrated L & H – provided another forum in which to continue to develop his outstanding virtues as a speaker. He became its auditor and gold medallist.

His friends included Francis Skeffington, better known today as Sheehy Skeffington, the name he adopted on marrying Hanna Sheehy, Arthur Clery, Constantine Curran, William Dawson, Colum, Gogarty and James Joyce. One must add the qualification that with Joyce friendship varied like the barometer. Herbert Gorman, his first biographer, shows us 'Joyce evasive, slightly withdrawn and coldly polite with Tom Kettle who had been magnified by university students into a second Parnell',[6] but in another mood Joyce admired Kettle and wrote a limerick:

> A holy Hegelian Kettle
> His faith which we cannot unsettle;
> If no one abused it
> He might have reduced it,
> But now he is quite on his mettle.[7]

Robert Lynd's description of Kettle as 'a young philosopher in a sad cloak' is indicative of changes wrought by the passage of a few years.[8] According to Constantine Curran, 'ill health interrupted his college terms and compelled him to retire to his father's farm or to Innsbruck and Switzerland'.[9] The nature of his illness has not been clearly stated but the evidence suggests that it was a form of nervous breakdown and that he was to have occasional recurrences.

If the cloud had a silver lining, it lay in the opportunities for rest cures abroad, even if these turned out to be something of a busman's holiday, perfecting his German and French and sitting under new masters. During a visit to Belgium he climbed the belfry of Mons and picked out the battlefields spread about it: Ligny, Fontenoy, Jemappes, Malplaquet. A Frenchman, similarly occupied, turned to him and voiced their unspoken thoughts, 'When will there be another?' They laughed the question away, believing it lacked reality.

JOURNALISM

Kettle took his BA in mental and moral science with second-class honours in 1902. In January 1903 he enrolled at the King's Inns to read law. He also became editor of *St Stephen's*, the university magazine, an honorary post bringing experience which must have been helpful when in the autumn of 1905, with the assistance of Skeffington, he became editor of *The Nationist*, a newly established and short-lived weekly review of Irish thought and affairs.

A tabloid of 16 pages or so, *The Nationist* sold for a penny. Each page contained a half-dozen or more articles, including at least one in Irish, a poem and a critique. Its poets were Padraic Colum, Thomas Keoghler, Joseph Campbell and Oliver Gogarty. It proposed to devote itself 'to criticism of contemporary life construed from the National point of view'. It supported the Parliamentary Party but did not propose to ignore 'what is fairly entitled the "Hungarian" policy and unfairly the "Sinn Féin" policy'. It supported the ideal of complete independence rather than Home Rule. It was in accord with the language movement and hoped to concern itself with industry and education.

Kettle's *Nationist* kept a critical eye on the Abbey Theatre but urged the public to support it. Padraic Colum's *The Land* was generously praised: 'Mr Colum has put on the stage the largest fact of Irish life; he has dramatised agrarianism, and written the secret history of emigration.'[10]

POLITICS

Meanwhile, Kettle had been elected president of the Young Ireland branch of the United Irish League, a 'ginger' group, generally called the 'YIBs', which hoped to combine the poetry of patriotism with the practical work of patriotism and to purify and harden the constitutional movement by bringing into it young, capable and enthusiastic men.

'The Philosophy of Politics' was the title of his inaugural address in the Mansion House in December 1905 and he displayed his flair as a speaker: 'Life is growth [he declared]; growth is change: and the one thing of which we are certain is that society must keep moving on. Freedom is a battle and a march. It has many bivouacs, but no barracks.'[11]

He condemned cynicism as the last treachery, the irredeemable defeat. 'After all,' said Kettle, 'there is the two-edged sword that will never fail you, with enthusiasm for one of its edges and irony for the other.'

We have become so accustomed to hearing politics decried and the state dismissed as soulless and uncaring that it is fascinating to encounter Kettle's luminous description of the state in action: 'And the State is the name by which we call the great human conspiracy against hunger and cold, against loneliness and ignorance; the State is the fostermother and warden of the arts, of love, of comradeship, of all that redeems from despair that strange adventure which we call human life.'[12]

His description of the novitiate through which in the politics of his day an idea passed before it became law also bears repetition:

It arises out of the misery, and contains in it the salvation of a countryside; the State welcomes it with a policeman's baton. It recovers; the State puts it in jail, on a plank bed, and feeds it on skilly. It becomes articulate in Parliament; a statesman from the moral altitude of £5,000 a year denounces it as the devilish device of a hired demagogue. It grows old, almost obsolete, no longer adequate; the statesman steals it, embodies it in an Act, and goes down to British history as a daring reformer.[13]

As Kettle matured, his charm and friendliness were appreciated far beyond his academic levels, bringing him into contact with every kind of Irishman, economists and manual workers, cattlemen and curates, labour leaders and market gardeners, track-runners, poets, county councillors and newspaper reporters. 'All these people, unknown to each other,' Constantine Curran recalled, 'had the same story to tell, not of a mere hail-fellow-well-met, but of unforced identity and comradeship. He spoke everyone's language without forsaking his own. All doors were open to him and he subjugated any chance company, not by his exceptional wit merely, but by fellowship.'[14]

One might have expected that a brilliant success lay ahead when he was called to the bar in April 1906, but fate decreed otherwise when he was invited to contest a by-election in East Tyrone. He may, in any case, have been temperamentally unsuited to legal practice and his essay 'Reveries of Assize' suggests that he was not enthralled by the process of law:

You had a sense of utter futility [he wrote] as you listened to the steady, infinitesimal drip of evidence. It was like the nagging and pecking patter of thin rain on a hat. It proved everything with absolute conclusiveness except the moral guilt of the prisoner. You have the same sense of the emptiness of criminology as a pale, sensitive face appears above the spikes of the dock. He might be a poet, an Assisi peasant turned saint, but certainly there is no signature of crime in his visage. As a matter of fact, he stabbed a neighbour to death because of a difference of opinion . . . [15]

The vacancy in East Tyrone was caused by the death of the Nationalist MP P.C. Doogan in June 1906 and Kettle held the seat by a narrow majority of 18 votes. In the fall of that year Kettle and another young Nationalist MP, Richard Hazelton, toured America as fund-raisers for the Irish Party. There was a reception in Carnegie Hall on 21 October and in the next few months Kettle spoke in many New England cities and the Middle West. His speeches were reported fairly by the *Irish World* but treated critically by the *Gaelic American*, the organ of the militant Clan na Gael.[16]

HOUSE OF COMMONS

When he delivered his maiden speech in the House of Commons on 2 May 1907 he complained that the Dublin police force was an Imperial and not a municipal concern, and really a branch of the Military Department which should be placed on the Army Estimates. It cost three times as much as the Sheffield police force.

In July 1907 he objected to the proposed grant to Lord Cromer on his retirement from Egypt. Speaking on behalf of what he called 'the oppressed and the outraged', he objected to 'this donation and dole to a retired despot'. He referred to an incident at Denshawi which resulted in four hangings, two life sentences and a number of long terms of imprisonment. 'Four hundred lashes were given to innocent Egyptians,' Kettle told the House, 'and we are asked to give Lord Cromer £50,000, which is a little more than £100 a lash.'[17]

At Westminster the leading orators included Asquith, Balfour and John Redmond. Before long, Kettle's increasingly large audiences were obliged to accept him as their equal. He was a born speaker, unlike those sometimes moved to eloquence by passionate conviction. John J. Horgan, who heard Kettle speak in the House of Commons, has left a graphic portrait of his former schoolfriend. 'Wit and humour, denunciation and appeal, paradox and epigram, gave point and effect to his fluent speeches. Tall and straight, with his soft handsome boyish face and bright eyes, he first startled and then compelled the attention of the House by his irresistible charm and luminous argument.'[18]

Kettle could be unforgivably caustic: 'Ulster Unionism is not a party. It is only an appetite. Take away from them the people who hope for office, the people who have canvassed for office for other people, and who are pushing the claims for office for their brothers and their brothers-in-law, and sons and nephews, and the Ulster Unionist party would be represented by about two members.'

He shone like a Sir Galahad in a debate on women's suffrage and accepted that in due course there would be women in parliament. 'Mr Speaker,' he drawled sardonically, 'they say that if we admit women the House will lose its intelligence – '. His sweeping gesture took in the packed benches. 'Mr Speaker, that is impossible.' The members roared with laughter. 'Mr Speaker, they tell me too', he continued, 'that the House will suffer in its morals. I don't believe that possible either.' Another gust of laughter acknowledged a double hit.

Kettle's support of the Irish Universities bill in 1908 is some-times regarded as his most useful contribution in parliament but it may well be that his criticism of the maladministration of the Old Age Pension Act in Ireland was more important.

The administration of the Act in Ireland had revealed acute and terrible poverty. The intentions of parliament, Kettle stressed, had been humane and generous but the Local Government Board's policy had been mean, niggardly and secret. Appeals were not heard in open court and decisions were made on undisclosed principles:

I say now this in conclusion [Kettle declared]. You have this Old Age Pension being administered in secret; you have pension officers who have been fined for disclosing to pension committees even a small part of the instructions upon which they act . . . We are not making any plea for the lax administration of the Act. For my part, I would rather see an old man or an old woman – harsh and full of temptation to poor people though it may be – I would rather see a poor man or a poor woman in Ireland, and I believe that the sense of the country would rather see them perish of hunger on the wayside than obtain one of your State pensions by a deliberate misrepresentation of facts or a deliberate lie.

Outside the House of Commons Kettle's duties included attendance at the council meetings of the United Irish League and at meetings organized by the League all over the country. He managed, too, to expand his connection in journalism and when James Joyce's collection of poems, *Chamber Music*, was published in 1907, Kettle reviewed it in the *Freeman's Journal*.

He praised it, crediting the best of the verses with 'the bright beauty of a crystal'. 'Mr Joyce's book', he concluded, 'is one that all his old friends will, with a curious pleasure, add to their shelves, and that will earn him many new friends.'[19]

Kettle's translation into English of Paul Dubois' *L'Irlande contemporaine* was published in Dublin and New York in 1908. 'Did you get the Dubois and is it as horrible as it seems to me?' he asked Alice Stopford Green, doubtless concealing an author's pride in his self-deprecatory question.

Tom Kettle married Mary Sheehy in the Pro-Cathedral on 8 September 1909. His bride was a daughter of David Sheehy MP and a niece of Father Eugene Sheehy, the so-called Land League priest. He had known her for a number of years, but as an unpaid Member of Parliament, a briefless barrister and an impecunious journalist, may have been too poor to wed. Now the situation was changed by his appointment as Professor of Economics in the newly formed National University.

The honeymoon, which he interrupted to make a fiery speech at the Young Egypt Congress in Geneva, was spent in Austria. On their return they lived at 23 Northumberland Road, where their only child, a daughter, was born in January 1913.

PROFESSOR OF ECONOMICS

When the House of Lords rejected the Budget in November 1909, the Liberals went to the country and when Tom Kettle contested East Tyrone in January 1910 as an Irish Nationalist, his instinctive command of the right phrase gained him an increased majority. 'Friends!' he saluted a welcoming party headed by a band and carrying torches. 'You have met us with God's two best gifts to man, fire and music.'

He appealed to the Protestants of the constituency to think for themselves. William of Orange was a Dutchman and he was dead. Was it worth quarrelling over a dead Dutchman?

Kettle's campaign was supported by Shane Leslie, the eldest son of Sir John Leslie of Glaslough, County Monaghan. He thought Kettle a delightful platform speaker, witty and lyrical. 'He could turn over weighty questions of economics or of international policy with an ease that struck home in the peasant mind.'

Kettle held his seat by a majority of 140. As the victor and Mrs Kettle drove away, Shane Leslie watched them admiringly. Kettle had the power to charm the House of Commons, a chair of economics and a beautiful wife. Leslie thought he had never seen a man more blessed. The baronet's son experienced envy mitigated by his knowledge of Kettle's sensitiveness, his prey to emotional distress and spiritual wrestlings. 'He was too brilliant to be happy, and his optimism and his pessimism seemed to keep house together.'[20]

We are nowadays so accustomed to seeing academics participate in politics that it comes as a surprise to find that many people, including Tom himself, believed that Professor Kettle could not do justice to the chair of economics if he remained in parliament. Because of this he withdrew from East Tyrone in December 1910 and this seat was taken by William Archer Redmond, a son of the leader of the Irish Parliamentary Party, in the December election.

Kettle's chair was not a prestigious one and his close friends and contemporaries did not take him altogether seriously in his new role. Arthur Clery has said, 'He certainly was not an economist'; William Dawson saw him as a dabbler in economics. Kettle's papers included notebooks containing drafts of lecture courses, the extent and detail of which show that he gave more time and thought to his subject than Clery and others would allow.

His class was small; in his first year he had only four students, one of whom was George O'Brien, who, until his death in 1973, spoke frequently of Kettle, who, on the sunny May afternoons, lectured, or rather talked, to his class under the trees in St Stephen's Green. For those who twitted him on the aridity of the dismal science, Professor Kettle had a ready answer.

If that is your experience of it blame the economists. For the slice of life, with which Economics has to deal, vibrates and, so to say, bleeds with human actuality. All science, all exploration, all history in its material factors, the whole epic of man's effort to subdue the earth and establish himself on it, fall within the domain of the economist.[21]

A judgment on Kettle's position as an economist is outside my scope but the late James Meenan, one of his successors, underlined the importance of his translation of Paul Dubois' *Contemporary Ireland* and praised his deeply humanistic approach.[22]

ESSAYIST

A collection of Kettle's essays, entitled *The Day's Burden*, was published in 1910 and provides eloquent testimony of a literary talent which political commitments prevented him from developing. Sheehy Skeffington found a review of Francis Thompson's *Health and Holiness* the gem of the book but my own favourite is a short essay, 'November First: The Day of All the Dead', which contains a description of autumn as Kettle must have seen it with a countryman's eye:

A wintry silence has fallen on the birds, if it be not for that epitome of loneliness, the cry of the lapwing, or the clangour of rooks or of wedged battalions of wild geese, cleaving the emptiness of the sky. Over all this ritual of desolation the trees prevail, towering above the rout like the captains of a defeated army. The flame of October has burned itself out; the glory of red and orange, and bronze which wrapped the woods in a conflagration of beauty has smouldered down to faint embers. The oak still keeps its leaf and here and there the eye encounters the bulk of an elm, not yet denuded . . .[23]

Kettle's introduction to Halévy's biography of Nietzsche contains some vibrant passages: 'That edged and glittering speech of his', Kettle wrote, 'owed much to his acknowledged masters, La Rochefoucauld, Voltaire, and Stendhal, the lapidaries of France. But it was something very intimately his own; he was abundantly dowered with the insight of malice, and malice always writes briefly and well. It has not the time to be obscure.'[24]

Kettle's literary gift, as I have mentioned, was evident in Clongowes. He contributed articles to *St Stephen's* and a number of his essays appeared in the *New Ireland Review*. He wrote professionally for the *Freeman's Journal* and contributed to the *Daily News* and other English papers. Eventually he earned a steady income as a freelance journalist.

He had the ability to encapsulate a personality in a phrase – of Isaac Butt he wrote, 'Butt should have been a god, and dwelt apart'; 'Parnell', he said, 'spoke like an invoice, definite to the third decimal point, and final' – and he could stir the imagination with generalizations.

Oratory . . . [he wrote] is complex, diffuse, netted beyond release in impermanent details. Its triumph is of the moment, momentary. The sound and rumour of great multitudes, passions hot as ginger in the mouth, torches, tumultuous comings and goings, and, riding through the whirlwind of it all, a personality, with something about him of the prophet, something of the actor, crying out not so much with his own voice as with that of his multitude and establishing with a gesture, refuting with a glance, stirring ecstasies of hatred and affection – [25]

What a pity that such a striking talent should have been occupied in writing pamphlets on the Old Age Pension Act and the economics of unionism!

Kettle said, 'Hell is paved with good epigrams,' but his own speech and writings were richly epigrammatic. 'If we are to believe at all we must believe in the future' – 'The Act of Union . . . made hope an absentee and enterprise an exile' – 'The open Secret of Ireland is that Ireland is a nation.' He defined a jingo as 'a man who pays for one seat in a tramcar and occupies two', and said, 'When in office the Liberals forget their principles and the Tories remember their friends.' He called optimism and pessimism the 'day and night of the human spirit'. His own utterances were deeply tinged with sombre colours. He said, 'Life is a cheap *table d'hôte* in a rather dirty restaurant, with time changing the plates before you have had enough of anything.' 'It is with ideas', he said, 'as with umbrellas, if left lying about they are peculiarly liable to a change of ownership.'

Kettle's own enthusiasm in literature included an admiration of G.K. Chesterton and he lectured in Cork in 1910 on the Chestertonian trilogy, *The Napoleon of Notting Hill*, *The Man who was Thursday* and *The Ball and the Cross*. He described Chesterton as a great navvy of letters. 'His only holiday from writing prose was to write verse, and when that palled he took up the frantic pencil which used to be his when he was an art student and diverted himself by illustrating a book or two, generally a novel of the great Catholic writer, Mr Hilaire Belloc.'

Belloc was a Liberal MP whom Kettle would have known at Westminster. 'I don't mind loquacity', he said, 'if it isn't Bello-quacity.'

Belloc's lines on a sundial:

> How slow the Shadow creeps: but when 'tis past
> How fast the Shadows fall. How fast! How fast!

serve as a reminder of how, at the opening of the second decade of the century, distant shadows menaced the existence of a host of young men and the more immediate class war threatened the leisure and privileges of the well-to-do.

In Dublin the drama centred on the confrontation of William Martin Murphy and Jim Larkin, which, in Horse Show Week 1913, led to the tram-men's strike and the lock-out.

The plight of Dublin's poor was highlighted by the collapse of two slum tenements in Church Street burying twenty in the rubble. There was serious rioting in Swords early in October when strikers tried to prevent cattle being taken to the Dublin market. Two loads of vegetables sent to market by P.J. Kettle were marked 'tainted goods'.

George Russell (AE) denounced the Shylocks of industry. 'If our Courts of Justice were Courts of Humanity,' he said, 'the masters of Dublin would be in the dock charged with criminal conspiracy.'[26] Tom Kettle was sufficiently broad-minded to see that there were faults on both sides. 'The ordinary Dublin employer', he said, 'is neither so big nor so bad as he appears in AE's stormy vision.'

His sympathies, however, were with the workers and he was one of those who founded a Peace Committee in an attempt to settle the strike. He knew that Dublin's wage levels were a scandal and when he thought of its housing, the spectre of Church Street rose before his eyes. 'As a Citizen of Dublin,' he wrote, 'I rend my garments and cry for forgiveness at the word. The mansion-slums of Dublin go as close as any material fact can go to a denial of the ways of God.'[27]

Meanwhile, in the sphere of national politics, Home Rule seemed assured. The bill had its third reading in January 1913 but Tom Kettle underestimated the significance of the rising belligerence of north-east Ulster.

He was a member of the Provisional Committee of the Irish Volunteers when that body was established in November 1913 at a meeting in the Rotunda. Incidentally when Larry Kettle rose to speak at that meeting, he was shouted down by trade unionists. P.J. Kettle and Andy Kettle, like other farmers, had employed scab labour to reap the harvest.

THE GREAT WAR

When war was declared in August 1914, Kettle was in Ostend buying arms for the Irish Volunteers. He remained in Belgium as war correspondent for the *Daily News* and described the German advance, the sacking of Louvain, the bombardment of Malines and the desecration of its great cathedral.

He visited the cathedral city and recorded his feelings in the newspaper:

I am not ashamed to confess that when I, an Irish Catholic, walked in to the Grand Place and saw the stamp of Berlin imprinted on those good grey walls I did not think at once of material injury, or money, or subscriptions. What came was anger against the desecration of a holy place. My mind said to me: 'This is how Nietzsche had, from his grave, spat, as he wished to spit, upon Nazareth.'[28]

Kettle, like Sir Philip Gibbs, for instance, could have become a leading war correspondent but he decided he would prefer to be a sixth-rate soldier than a first-rate man of letters. He was commissioned in the Dublin Fusiliers in November 1911 and, because of his poor health and gift of oratory, he was kept in Ireland as a recruiting agent.

Home Rule had meanwhile received the royal assent, its implementation postponed until after the war by a Suspensory Act. John Redmond had reaffirmed his pledge of support for England at Woodenbridge, County Wicklow, in a speech which split the Volunteers into the Irish Volunteers, led by Eoin MacNeill, and the National Volunteers loyal to Redmond.

For Kettle the invasion of Belgium was a crime against civilization. 'The Blood-and-Ironmongers have entered into possession of the soul of humanity.' The political thought of Germany had been corrupted for a generation. 'It has been foul with the odour of desired shambles.' He accepted unquestioningly that England would honour the Home Rule agreement: 'Here, at the opening of this vast and bloody epic, Great Britain is right with the conscience of Europe. It is assumed that she has reconciled Ireland. A reconciled Ireland is ready to march side by side with her to any desperate trial.'

As an undergraduate, he had conducted an anti-recruiting campaign during the Boer War but now Lieutenant Kettle went up and down the country urging enlistment. 'Nowadays', he said, ' the absentee is the man who stays at home.'

He wrote blatantly martial Kiplingesque verses:

> We ain't no saints or scholars much, but fightin' men and clean,
> We've paid the price, and three times thrice for Wearin' o' the Green
> We held our hand out frank and fair, and half forgot Parnell,
> For Ireland's hope and England's too – and it's yours to save or sell.
> For it's Paddy this, and Paddy that, 'Who'll stop the Uhlan blade?'
> But Tommy Fitz from Malahide, and Monaghan's McGlade,
> When the ranks are set for judgment, lads, and the roses droop and fade,
> It's Ireland in the firin' line! when the price of God is paid.[29]

EASTER 1916

When an unexpected rebellion erupted at Easter 1916, some patriotic Irishmen wearing uniforms were placed in a quandary. Was it their duty to oppose the insurgents? Lord Dunsany, a serving soldier, was shot and wounded while making his way to join an army group. James Connolly was the victim of a marksman of the Royal Irish Regiment. Kettle, according to Robert Lynd, 'fought in the streets of Dublin' to suppress the rebellion.[30] The evidence for this statement is shadowy and William Fallon quotes Kettle as saying, 'The circumstances are so peculiar that one doesn't know which side one ought to join.'[31] Perhaps, like Surgeon Tobin of St Vincent's Hospital, who ventured to advise the rebels in St Stephen's Green though armed with nothing more lethal than a blackthorn stick, he made a verbal protest. But he is reported to have been taken before Countess Markievicz, who spoke to him rudely and ordered his detention.[32] This unreliable report is referred to in the Preface. It was L. J. Kettle who was detained.

He certainly saw the Easter Rising as madness, destructive to the efforts of parliamentary nationalism, but when the executions transformed the apparently futile gesture, he was moved to indignation and pity. 'These men will go down to history as heroes and martyrs,' he said, 'and I will go down – if I go down at all – as a bloody British officer.'

Meeting J.F. Byrne (Cranly in Joyce's *A Portrait of the Artist as a Young Man*), he told him that he had applied to the commanding officer at the Curragh to be sent to France on active service.

THE BATTLE OF THE SOMME

Events of 1 July 1916 in Picardy were described by an Irish doctor serving in an RAMC casualty-clearing station:

At 6 o'clock the most deafening bombardment arose; the air simply quivered ... and then at 7 o'clock dead silence, or what seemed like it (I was two miles back). After that a low roar; the Hun's machine guns and shrapnel were at work. We knew our men were up and over the parapet. We back there could only wonder how things went ... We heard the Hun's shrapnel and machine guns. Nothing, one would think, could live in such a fire; but two hours later we were told our men have all the first line trench, are held at one spot but are advancing to right and left. What 'held' meant at such a time in such a fire we realised. We all had friends in it.[33]

It was in this inferno, the Battle of the Somme, that Kettle was destined to die. He left Dublin on 14 July. By then it was clear that the British assault had not gained the expected rapid victory. Presumably Lieutenant Kettle went to a camp where a 'rough, commando type training' was given to men who had not been under fire before going to his regimental base. And soon he experienced the horrors of trench warfare.

As a war-correspondent, Kettle had described the conflict as a hell of suffering. 'And through it, over its flaming coals, Justice must walk, were it on bare feet.' Kettle the combatant found himself wading in a quagmire of mud, a glutinous estuary of ravaged earth, where now and then his squelching footsteps found firmer purchase on submerged bodies of the recent dead. He submitted to privations which reduced him physically but refused to go on sick leave and turned down a posting to a staff appointment.

Enjoying a respite behind the front line, he had time to write to Dublin. 'The Sinn Féin nightmare upset me a little . . . ', he admitted. 'We took the side of justice, we did the right thing, we helped to bring the North and South together . . . '.[34]

Towards the end of August his battalion was ordered to the rising sector north of the Somme where battle raged for possession of Longueval, Delville Wood, Guillemont and Ginchy. On 3 September Guillemont was taken. Philip Gibbs has described the astonishing impetuosity of the Irish troops – 'They went forward with their pipes playing them on, in a wild irresistible assault.' A captain of the Munsters planted a green flag with a yellow harp in the centre of the pulverized village.[35]

Next day Kettle wrote the celebrated sonnet, 'To my Daughter Betty':

> In wiser days, my darling rosebud, blown
> To beauty proud as was your Mother's prime.
> In that desired, delayed, incredible time,
> You'll ask why I abandoned you, my own,
> And the dear heart that was your baby throne,
> To dice with death. And oh! they'll give you rhyme
> And reason: some will call the thing sublime,
> And some decry it in a knowing tone.
> So here, while the mad guns curse overhead,
> And tired men sigh with mud for couch and floor,
> Know that we fools, now with the foolish dead,
> Died not for flag, nor King, nor Emperor,
> But for a dream, born in a herdsman's shed,
> And for the secret Scripture of the poor.[36]

Heavy German shelling killed 200 men and seven officers and, having assumed command of B company, Kettle received orders on 8 September to move before Ginchy at midnight. Saturday, 9 September was beautiful but misty. At headquarters, in the presence of the Prime Minister, Herbert Asquith, who was visiting the Somme, Sir Henry Rawlinson, commander of the British Fourth Army, waited expectantly while an intense preliminary bombardment proceeded.[37]

The taking of Ginchy has been described as the 'hottest thing' since the landing at Suvla Bay. 'From a non-military, untechnical, human point of view,' Philip Gibbs wrote, 'the greatness of the capture of Ginchy is in the valour of those Irish boys who . . . went straight on to the winning posts like Irish race-horses.'

Many failed to complete the race. At the sound of the whistle at 4.45 p.m. Kettle led his company over the parapet into no man's land. He fell almost immediately, shot through the chest by a sniper. Emmet Dalton, who was following, saw that he was dying and pressed a crucifix into his hand. His body was not recovered and his name is inscribed on the Memorial to the Missing at Thiépval.

AFTERMATH

Tom Kettle remains a tragic and largely forgotten victim of Irish nationalism. 'I think nobody can deny that he was betrayed,' G.K. Chesterton said, 'but it was not by the English soldiers with whom he marched to war, but by those very English politicians with whom he sacrificed so much to remain at peace.'[38] What was clear to GKC has remained less evident to many of Kettle's fellow countrymen, to whom green rather than khaki is seen as the preferred wear for 1916 and to have died in Dublin more honourable than death on the Western Front.

W.B. Yeats's poem 'An Irish Airman Foresees His Death' lacked the myth-making force of the superb 'Easter 1916' – *our part/To murmur name upon name . . .* The thousands of Irish ex-servicemen who crowded into Dublin's Mansion House on 16 July 1919 are nameless. All we know is that they decided not to join a victory march to be held three days later. On the platform, Mrs Kettle seconded a motion to boycott it. 'Did any Irish nationalist fight for any country except the country of his birth?' she asked. But they were directed to march past their former House of Parliament saluting Lord French not as an Irish soldier but as Lord Lieutenant and representing an executive responsible for the betrayal of the Irish nationalists who fought and fell in the war.

Edward Martyn once responded to a complaint of flogging in the navy by saying that Irishmen who join the army or navy of England deserved to be flogged but he had his tongue in his cheek, wishing to annoy the members of the Kildare Street Club. The flak of recent Remembrance Sundays, nevertheless, confirms a prevailing ambivalence in this regard. Tom Kettle would have deplored this narrowness. He said prophetically: 'My only counsel to Ireland is, that in order to become deeply Irish, she must become European.'[39]

NOTES

1. Andrew J. Kettle, *Material for Victory*, Laurence J. Kettle (ed.) (Dublin 1958), *passim*.

2. Oliver St John Gogarty, *It Isn't This Time of Year At All* (London 1954), p. 20. See also Anthony Quinn, 'Flanders' Fields and Irish Recollections' (*Capuchin Annual* [1977], 342–3) and 'But for a Dream' (*The Cross* [1977], 67: 25–6).
3. *Clongownian* (1896), 1: 18–20.
4. Oliver St John Gogarty, *Start from Somewhere Else* (New York 1955), p. 76.
5. Padraic Colum, 'Tom Kettle, A Memory', *Dublin Magazine* (1949), 24: 28–35.
6. Herbert Gorman, *James Joyce* (London 1941).
7. Cited by Constantine Curran in *James Joyce Remembered* (New York 1968), p. 76.
8. Robert Lynd, *If the Germans Conquered England* (London 1917), p. 137.
9. C.P. Curran, *Under the Receding Wave* (Dublin 1970), p. 141.
10. *The Nationist*, 5 October 1905.
11. *The Day's Burden: Studies, Literary & Political and Miscellaneous Essays* (Dublin 1937), p. 7.
12. *Ibid.*, p. 16.
13. *Ibid.*, p. 15.
14. Curran, *op. cit.*, p. 146.
15. *The Day's Burden*, p. 59.
16. For greater detail see J.B. Lyons, *The Enigma of Tom Kettle* (Dublin 1983), pp. 86–108.
17. Kettle's words in parliament are taken from *Hansard*.
18. John J. Horgan, *From Parnell to Pearse* (Dublin 1948), p. 202.
19. *Freeman's Journal*, 1 June 1907.
20. Shane Leslie, *ibid.*, 3 November 1916.
21. *The Day's Burden*, p. 129.
22. James Meenan, *George O'Brien* (Dublin 1980); see also Introduction to *The Day's Burden* (Dublin 1968).
23. *The Day's Burden* (1937), p. 197.
24. Introduction to J.M. Hone's translation of Daniel Halévy's *Life of Friedrich Nietzsche* (London 1911).
25. Tom Kettle (ed.), *Irish Orators and Oratory* (Dublin 1915), p. ix.
26. *Freeman's Journal*, 3 November 1913.
27. *Ibid.*, 24 September 1913.
28. *The Ways of War* (London 1917), p. 111.
29. *Poems & Parodies* (Dublin 1916), p. 77.
30. Robert Lynd, *op. cit.*, p. 139.
31. William Fallon: in Curran papers UCD.
32. Maurice Headlam, *Irish Reminiscences* (London 1947), p. 175.
33. Anon. 'The Great Offensive Picardy, July 1916', *Dublin Journal of Medical Science* (1916), 142: 195–9.
34. Kettle papers – see J.B. Lyons, *op. cit.*, p. 308.
35. Philip Gibbs, *The Germans on the Somme* (London 1917).
36. *Poems & Parodies*, p. 15.
37. A.H. Farrar-Hockley, *The Somme* (London 1983), p. 224.
38. G.K. Chesterton, *Irish Impressions* (London 1919), p. 170.
39. *The Day's Burden* (1937), p. xii.

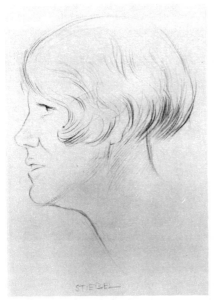

10. Helen Waddell by Helen Stiebel (From *The Bookman*, December 1933)

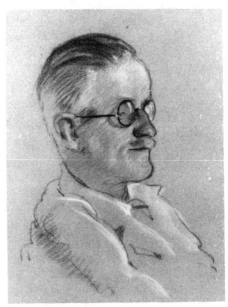

11. James Joyce by Sean O'Sullivan (Courtesy of the National Gallery of Ireland)

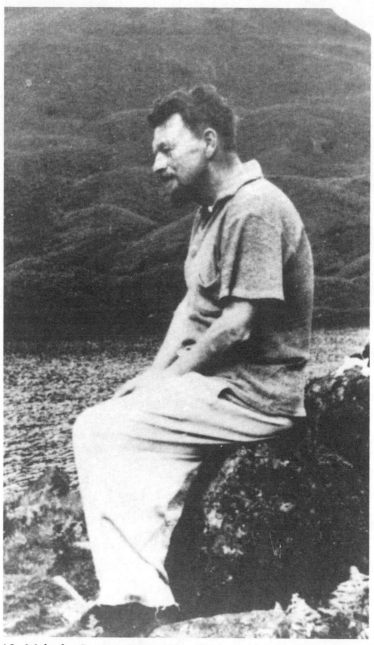

12. Malcolm Lowry, June 1957 (Courtesy of the University of
British Columbia)

10

Helen Waddell:
The Irish Dimension

I

HELEN Waddell described her father as 'the Vicar of Wakefield turned Chinese scholar'. One of her early memories was of his voice on the verandah of their Tokyo bungalow just after dawn murmuring the psalms in Hebrew, the New Testament in Greek and the Lord's Prayer in Japanese.[1] His gift of tongues was to be her own golden inheritance and *The Wandering Scholars* the most enduring expression of her linguistic genius.

The youngest of a family of ten children, Helen Jane Waddell was born on 31 May 1889 in Tokyo, where her father was a Presbyterian missionary. The Rev. Hugh Waddell was a Belfast man; his wife, Jane Martin, came from County Down. Despite her mother's death in 1891 and her father's remarriage, for the protection of his family, to Martha Waddell, a middle-aged cousin, her Japanese childhood was idyllic. She enjoyed the interplay of reality and make-believe that is childhood's priceless endowment. The great Buddha of Kamakura was a colossal object which a missionary's child could learn to venerate. She shared secrets with the snakes and lizards and at eight years of age her closest friend was a toad who lived under the verandah and never moved. His stillness fascinated her, as she recalled: 'He was older than the other toads, and perhaps he was stiff . . . No one knew where his hole was. He had never been seen going or coming: he was squat and motionless, or else he was not.'[2]

Adolescence followed in Belfast when it finally dawned on Hugh Waddell that his two daughters deserved a conventional education. Their brothers had been sent off in pairs, long before, to Campbell College. Four of them studied medicine, two entered

the ministry and Sam Waddell was the successful playwright
Rutherford Mayne.

Meg and Helen attended the Victoria College for Girls. Their
education was not interrupted by their father's death in 1901 for
the dutiful older brothers met their expenses. The elder sister's
regular tuition had been so delayed that she was satisfied to take
a pass BA, RUI. She then married the Rev J.D. Martin and
settled happily at Kilmacrew House, an old-world residence in
County Down.

Helen entered the newly established Queen's University in
1908 with a scholarship awarded *summa cum laude* and was joined
there in 1910 by her close friend Maude Clarke, a future Oxford
history don. They were to collaborate in 1915 in writing a novel,
Discipline, which was sent to many publishers without acceptance.
Meanwhile, Helen's altogether exceptional ability and originality
had been noted by her examiners. She took the BA with first-
class honours in 1911, proceeding MA with a thesis on 'Milton,
the Epicurist' in 1912.

Openings for brilliant women graduates were few in number
and Gregory Smith, Helen's professor, was an avowed anti-
feminist, quite determined to choose a male assistant though
convinced of her outstanding qualities. It says something for her
equable temperament and lack of pugnacity that she remained
devoted to Professor Smith. But in any case she conceived it to
be her duty to stay at home with her ailing stepmother, a
depressed and difficult woman and a secret drinker.

By then four of her brothers were medical practitioners but
Dr Billy Waddell, who graduated in Edinburgh in 1909, was a
drug abuser. Helen had been Billy's close companion in their
Tokyo adventures until he was sent to Campbell College and she
remembered him as having 'an ugly mouth and the most beautiful smile I ever saw'; Billy was an odd mixture 'of sensuousness and
imagination, spirit and flesh, religion and devilry'. She was twenty-
two when she realized the misfortune that had befallen him.

Billy went into a private mental hospital for treatment but
could not stand the grim surroundings. Helen wrote quite optimistically to her sister. 'You needn't be afraid of his going back
to the drug. I was talking to him by himself for a bit, and he
speaks of it with a kind of a shudder, says he is glad, *so* glad, to be

cured . . . We'll have to pray for him desperately but I'm in great heart about him.'[3]

The young doctor wished to join the Indian Medical Service but instead went to sea as a ship's surgeon and was washed overboard in a storm. Another brother, newly ordained in the Presbyterian ministry, died unexpectedly from a heart complaint six months later.

The picture of Helen Waddell on the dust-jacket of Dame Felicitas Corrigan's biography depicts a plain-faced young woman, a prototype, perhaps, for Dorothy Parker's catty epigram: 'Men seldom make passes / At girls who wear glasses.' Her warm personality and lively intellect more than compensated for anything she lacked in looks and the boys at Queen's found her entrancing.

Her admirers included two medical students, Brice Clarke, a brother of her friend Maude, and Billy Lynd (the essayist's brother), who proposed to her regularly and was regularly rejected. Dr Lynd joined the Cunard Line as ship's surgeon and she corresponded with him but when on leave in 1917 he told her he was engaged to a girl he met on the *Caronia* and she had the good grace to feel jealous. Poor Lynd was widowed within a year of his marriage and they resumed their friendship. Then Dr Brice Clarke MC turned up in 1919 to express his love in phrases like 'broken bits of Donne and the *Laus Veneris*, and *The Last Ride Together*'.[4]

Other wooers sought her hand, one of whom – she called him 'the Mourne Mountains man' – almost did persuade her to marry him, but through some psychological quirk, possibly Freudian in nature, her deepest friendships were with married men or widowers a good deal older than herself. One of these, Professor George Saintsbury of Edinburgh, whom she met when he came to Belfast as extern examiner, corresponded with her regularly until his death at a great age in 1933. Another, the Rev. George Taylor, the missionary founder and headmaster of a school in India, was a genuine father-figure but human enough to resent Saintsbury's admiration. He supplied her with books and money in her penurious twenties.

While engaged as Isabella Tod Memorial Scholar in a study of 'Women as a Dramatic Asset', a study which had not fired her imagination, she idly leafed through a collection of Chinese classics that had been in the house for years. James Legge, some-

time missionary and later professor of Chinese at Oxford, supplied
literal translations and challenged readers to transmute his prose
into verse. Memories of the East ignited Helen's creativity; within
days she had a sheaf of lyrics that even Professor Gregory Smith
agreed were good.

   Her luminous words describe a mandarin's garden:

> Peach blossom after rain
> Is deeper red;
> The willow fresher green;
> Twittering overhead;
> And fallen petals lie wind-blown
> Unswept upon the court-yard stone.[5]

   Certain Chinese customs make for heartbreak, as when a bride
finds that decorum forbids her to visit her family home:

> How say they that the Ho is wide,
> When I could ford it if I tried?
> How say they Sung is far away
> When I can see it every day?
>
> Yet must indeed the Ho be deep
> When I have never dared the leap;
> And since I am content to stay
> Sung must indeed be far away.[6]

   Lyrics from the Chinese was accepted by Constable and published
in 1913. *The Irish Booklover* noted that Helen Waddell's first book
had 'won warm eulogiums from the critics'. Her two-act play,
The Spoiled Buddha, was produced in the Grand Opera House,
Belfast, in February 1915 (and published by Dublin's Talbot
Press in 1919). Her literary career was launched and she was
writing children's stories but the splash was not a great one and
she was conscious of how well Maude Clarke was doing at
Oxford and that another friend, Cathleen Nesbitt, was a rising
Shakespearean actress.

   George Saintsbury, by then a gallant of seventy-five, sent a
charming greeting for her thirtieth birthday:

> A ta trentième
> O ma Lointaine
> Princesse,
> Moi, je t'adore
> Bien plus encore
> Sans cesse.[7]

Alas! the princess remained the prisoner of a demanding, if not actually wicked, stepmother whom she had almost come to hate, or more accurately the captive of her own sense of duty and love. She never forgot that Martha had once been tender and motherly. 'I think I'd have been starved for love', she reminded her sister, 'if I hadn't had her when I was little.'[8]

Mrs Waddell died on 25 June 1920. Some days later Helen wrote to Saintsbury from Kilmacrew: 'It's wet, and the candle is blowing at the open window and there's a corncrake out in the dark. And I've felt human again for the first time. My mother died last Friday in her sleep. I found her in the chair.'[9]

II

Dazed by events, Helen rested at Kilmacrew, her securest haven. She let the Belfast house and set off for Oxford in the fall. She enrolled at Somerville College as a Ph.D. candidate, living in rooms in Keble Road. She supplemented her funds by correcting examination papers and, appointed to a lectureship under the Cassell Trust Fund in 1921, gave eight lectures on 'Mime in the Middle Ages'. These were rapturously received. Her voice filled the room and she had inherited her father's effortless oratory.

Nevertheless, she was unsettled at Oxford, impatient of academic restrictions, too old to be awed by the prospect of a doctorate. 'I'm horribly afraid that artists and journalists are more my sort than academic people,' she confided to Saintsbury. She did not complete the required terms of residence but applied unsuccessfully for some quite unsuitable posts. Then in 1923, after many disappointments and false starts, Helen, in her biographer's words, was 'suddenly presented with the golden key that fitted into the hidden door opening into the landscape of her dreams'.[10] This was her election by the Council of Lady Margaret Hall to the Susette Taylor Travelling Fellowship, which provided £200 annually for two years, enabling her to attend the Sorbonne and read at the Bibliothèque Nationale.

For Helen, steeped in the literature of the Middle Ages, the streets of Paris were thronged with ghosts of past centuries; so much so that when admitted with fever to the Pasteur Hospital by Doctor Vaudremer, her creative mind, throughout a long sleepless night, exchanged her identity for that of the hapless Héloïse.

Returning to London in 1925, Helen continued her work in the reading-room of the British Museum and took a small flat in Ormonde Terrace, Primrose Hill. *The Wandering Scholars* was accepted by Constable and published in April 1927. Its success was immediate and a third edition was required in December. The notice in *The Times* is representative of the literary pages' enthusiasm. '*The Wandering Scholars* comes from the mind of a scholar and the graceful pen of a wit . . . unlike certain sapless professorial commentaries, her discoveries are both exciting and charming.'[11] The Royal Society of Literature gave Helen the A.C. Benson Medal, the first time the award was made to a woman. 'She writes about poetry absolutely unknown to me', Walter de la Mare remarked to the publisher, 'in a fashion that is itself poetry.' She was elected to the fellowship of the Royal Literary Society in 1928.

The commentary in *The Wandering Scholars* is, indeed, an extended lyric but it also succeeded in creating an appetite for more which Helen's next book, *Mediaeval Latin Lyrics*, was designed to satisfy. Its publication in 1929 enhanced her reputation and consolidated her position in London's literary and social life.

If those books were caviar to the general, *Peter Abelard*, the novel, published in 1933, was a popular success. Within fifteen years 85,000 copies were sold and it was translated into many languages. Her royalties enabled her to buy a house in London but the care and maintenance of this establishment at 32 Primrose Hill Road ate into her time, as AE (George Russell) had warned her it would. *Beasts and Saints* was published in 1934, *The Desert Fathers* in 1936 and there were other minor works, including her essay on John of Salisbury, whom she bore no grudge for his part as intermediary between Hadrian and Henry when Ireland was granted to the latter by the pope in 1155. She does not, indeed, mention that political engagement, being more concerned with the position of John the humanist, driven back to France by the King's displeasure.

Thirty years before he had stood in the schools, *admodum adolescens*, hardly more than a boy, greedy for every word that fell from the lips of Abelard, one of the last to hear the great voice, before it fell abruptly silent: behold him again on the Petit Pont, the crowds again about him, the old familiar arguments, the dear disputes. 'Happy the exile, to which such place is given!'[12]

Helen Waddell experienced little of the tetchiness that Irish reviewers commonly reserve for their Irish contemporaries. The *Irish Statesman*'s reviewer ('L.R.') admitted that he was not sufficiently knowledgeable to do justice to the book. He would have returned it were it not simply too good to let go. He praised its 'beautiful warm style', its 'immense scholarship' without the mark of either pedant or popularizer. 'What has happened is that Miss Waddell's gaze, bent for years on crabbed medieval manuscripts puzzling out deletion and palimpsest, has never frozen into the scholar's stare. It has always kept human, kept its sense of beauty, its sense of fun, its sense of tragedy.'[13] *Studies* found her translations 'marvellously happy in their reproduction of the spirit and flavour of the originals'.[14]

Gerard Murphy's notice of *Mediaeval Latin Lyrics* in *The Irish Statesman* praised the book for bringing 'a wealth of pleasing literature within the range of those who know no Latin, and not infrequently discovering to the Latinist beauties which he might otherwise have passed by unnoticed'. Even fully-fledged classicists capable of reading the originals quite readily would gain a truer appreciation of Ausonius's lines on the Moselle at evening from Helen's rendering:

> What colour are they now, thy quiet waters?
> The evening star has brought the evening light,
> And filled the river with the green hillside;
> The hill-tops waver in the rippling water,
> Trembles the absent vine and swells the grape
> In thy clear crystal.

He calls this poem, written without adding or omitting a word, 'a poem which rivals the exquisite hexameters of the original in delicate rhythms and suggestiveness'.[15]

Dr J.S. Crone, editor of *The Irish Booklover*, also praised *Mediaeval Latin Lyrics* but a few years later 'G.M.' (presumably Gerard Murphy), reviewing Jack Lindsay's *Medieval Latin Poets*, did not resist the temptation to compare Lindsay's rendering of certain poems with Helen's and, in the instances he cited, seemed inclined to give the palm to Lindsay. This stringent critic wondered if it would have been preferable to render the Latin into English prose.

Many of the Latin poems translated by both authors are pleasing in themselves, quite apart from the knowledge they give us about the thoughts and emotions

of men of a past age. The same could be said of a few only of Miss Waddell's
translations, and of still fewer of Mr Lindsay's. Where Miss Waddell and Mr
Lindsay have failed others are not likely to be successful.[16]

Helen could hardly quarrel with what was an expression of
opinion but on reading T.B. Rudmose-Brown's review of *Peter
Abelard* she bridled and despatched a letter to Seumas O'Sullivan,
editor of the *Dublin Magazine*: 'I am a little aggrieved,' she complained. 'I wrote what I thought was a novel and Professor
Rudmose-Brown reviews it as if it were a monograph on
scarabs.' She countered the critic's most frequent query – 'On
what evidence?' – by insisting on her licence as a novelist to
invent providing she had not invented anything contradictory to
actual fact.[17]

Rudmose-Brown's probing questions permitted a parade of
his own learning. Was Alberic of Rheims, he asked, a teacher
there at the period of Miss Waddell's story? Gerbert did not
study 'Arabic and geometry at the schools of the Saracens'. There
is an absurd misprint on page 119 six lines from the bottom,
capital H for small h.

She answered the Trinity College don point by point until her
shining scholarship left that of her 'generous reviewer', as she
called him, suspect. Yes, Alberic may well have taught at Rheims
at the period in question. Rudmose-Brown has 'not quite accurately remembered' what Manutuis has said about it. The twelfth
century believed that Gerbert had studied Arabic; the revelations
of modern scholarship are irrelevant. The upper-case letter on
page 119 was *intended*. The critic has failed to understand the
sentence in which Abelard prays 'that God would save him from
Himself' (upper-case letter).

For a man to pray to be saved from himself [lower case letter] is common
enough . . . But there is another state of mind, less rational, less frequent, but
agonising, that would pray to be saved from God, 'Lest having Thee, to have
naught else beside'. John Donne would have understood it when he wrote his
Litany, and St Augustine, and the writer of the 139th Psalm: 'Whither shall I
flee from Thy presence? . . . if I make my bed in hell, behold Thou art there.'

Then, tongue in cheek, she acknowledged her critic's 'mag-
nanimity' and bowed out, leaving the discomfited professor to
indulge in the difficult exercise of saving face while beating a full
retreat.

The Desert Fathers was reviewed by Padraic Colum, who observed that what knowledge most readers have of the monks of the desert derives from Anatole France's *Thaïs* or from the pages of Gibbon or Lecky, men who 'were incapable of understanding the spirit back of them'. But Helen Waddell – 'whose work adds not only to our knowledge but to our imagination' – in her translations of the sayings of the Fathers brings before us 'men of judgement, wisdom, deep humanity. Around those sayings flows the silence of the desert; they are as if spoken after a long period of silence.'[18]

Her selections reflect her humility, charity and sense of humour: 'An old man said "there is no stronger virtue than to scorn no man . . . ".' The monk Serapion explained why he sold the only gospel he possessed: 'I sold that same word that ever used to say to me "sell what thou hast and give to the poor".'[19]

Beasts and Saints, which devotes a chapter to Ciaran, Kevin, Brendan and other Irish saints, was noticed by 'Colm' in the *Irish Booklover*. 'This is surely the most delightful *féirín* ever available to doting parents for birthday use or indeed as a gift for any grown-up not too sophisticated to read of saints and wonders.' The simplicity of the original tales was retained in the translations. 'But how perfect it is, how exact her choice of words and how reverent, too, in spite of the twinkling humour that can laugh at holy things. Ireland may take pride in Helen Waddell, for her true following in the Seanchaí tradition.'[20]

To be grouped with the Seanchaí was a well-meant but doubtful compliment to a scholar of Helen Waddell's erudition, nor can that limiting label, Anglo-Irish poet, be readily attached to one whose life and work had a wider, international context. And yet, throughout her writings, there is unquestionably an Irish dimension. This is clearest in her own verses, such as those lines that sprang into her mind, unbidden, on her return to London after a visit to Kilmacrew:

> I shall not go to heaven when I die,
> But if they let me be,
> I think I'll take a road I used to know
> That goes by Shere-na-garagh and the sea . . .[21]

It is lightly concealed in the novel, *Peter Abelard*, a veritable palimpsest in which the events of a celebrated love-story are written across a background of patristic scholarship and ecclesiastical intrigue. The tale opens in the narrow streets of twelfth-century Paris but Irish embellishments are nonchalantly added; the woods and waters of Brittany are indistinguishable from those of County Down. One of Malachy's ascetic monks from Armagh, faint from a prolonged Lenten fast, makes a welcome change from the common, roistering Irish stereotype. The perfectly balanced inscriptions on the vellum page of the little nun, Godric, never lost a distinctive Irish character in the fashioning of certain letters. Denise, in whose welcoming household Héloïse finds sanctuary and comfort when bearing Abelard's child, is an undisguised and loving portrait of Helen Waddell's sister, Meg Martin. The little fleet of ducks which at evening Héloïse called from the river were Ulster ducks; the 'snipe drumming on the bog' were birds Helen had heard drumming in the peat bog behind Kilmacrew House. And the book closes with St Columbanus's gloss on a missal at Bóbbio: 'By whose grief our wound was healed: by whose ruin our fall was stayed.'

Peter Abelard was one of three books short-listed for the Harmsworth Award by the Irish Academy of Letters' reading committee. The final adjudication by the English poet laureate, John Masefield, gave the prize to Lord Dunsany's *The Curse of the Wise Woman*.

Her books of Latin lyrics are peopled by celebrities such as Virgil and Petronius Arbiter but one finds several Irishmen there too, Columbanus, Colman the Irishman, and Sedulius, a Latinized form of Sheil. Columbanus was austere but she portrays a softer side: 'squirrels came and sat on his shoulder and ran in and out of his cowl . . . and when Valery the gardener at Luxeuil came into his classroom and brought the smell of roses with him, Columbanus would stop in his lecture to cry, "Nay then, it is thou, beloved, who art lord and abbot of this monastery." '[22]

The birthplace of Sedulius Scottus is unknown. She pictures him arriving in Liège *c.* 840 with two rain-sodden companions. When they sought sanctuary as clerics in holy orders at the bishop's house, they were welcomed and Sedulius was appointed *scholasticus* in the cathedral schools.

Some contemporary of Sedulius may have transcribed that Priscian manuscript 'snatched up and safe' in the wallet of an Irish scholar fleeing a Viking raid and taken by him to Cologne for later transfer to St Gall, where it still remains, having escaped destruction by the Huns.

When a group of Irish pilgrims, returning from Rome, had halted at St Gall *c.* 850, two of them, Marcellus, 'a mighty scholar both in classics and divinity', and his elderly uncle, Bishop Marcus, were persuaded to stay. Their decision annoyed the other pilgrims. 'Old Marcus came down to the courtyard, wearing his stole, to bless them, and watch them make their slow way down the pass and follow them with the eyes of the mind across France to the valley of the Loire and so to Nantes, or through Germany and the Low Countries, there to take ship for home.' Their departure did not bother Marcellus, intent on his studies. 'But the bishop was an old man; the Alps were not so friendly as the blue Wicklow hills, and though he never reached Ireland again he seems to have left "the nest that Irishmen built" to live in quiet "a holy man", says Heric of Auxerre at St Medard.' [23]

Helen praised Oliver Goldsmith ('always soft-hearted to the discredited') for supporting generations of disinterested scholars in *An Enquiry into the Present State of Polite Learning in Europe*, albeit many of them 'generally carried on a petty traffic in some little creek . . . '.

III

Established in London, Helen Waddell showed goodwill towards Irish writers. 'By the way,' she wrote to Seumas O'Sullivan, 'I'm what they call "adviser" to Constable now, and they are uncommonly well disposed to Irish writers. Will you bear that in mind, for yourself and any friends you have?'[24] But in the event she was obliged to send him the publisher's familiar refrain: 'All poetry is terribly hard to sell, but collected editions the hardest of all.'[25]

Her introduction to W.F. Marshall's *Ballads and Verses from Tyrone* (1929) admits a partiality for a certain kind of verse: 'You cannot follow the drums to *vers libre*, nor keep time to it with your fists on the table and your feet on the floor, nor dance to it in a loft.' She could see the resemblance between old 'Congo' Maguire, the hero of one of Marshall's ballads, and the harum-scarum Archpoet featured in *Wandering Scholars* – 'He died in the workhouse in January, very much as the Archpoet did in St Martin's cloister in Cologne.'[26]

She was devoted to AE. He encouraged her when she was writing *Peter Abelard* and said, 'I could not bear George Moore's tampering with the tale. He was not equal to imagining so much passion and beauty.'[27] Helen also had avoided reading Moore's *Héloïse and Abélard* 'lest that wizard prose of his should come between me and these two so sharply remembered in my own mind . . .'. [28] When AE read her novel, he sensed that she had lived the part of Héloïse. 'It's not only by vision we revisit the past; our hearts may sink into it and know what others have known.'[29]

He warned her against the dangers of social success. 'You watch or you will become nothing but a handshake and a brilliant talker, like James Stephens – that was what ruined him.'[30] His self-drawn Christmas card after the publication of *Beasts and Saints* depicted 'A Lion meditating in the desert after partaking of a saint. Notice God-given halo.' On the back of the card he wrote: 'Forgive me for petulance about Saints. They are too much with us in Ireland, and I forget that elsewhere some might deserve the name.'[31]

She lunched with AE in December 1933 and later in the month with George Bernard Shaw – 'I feel rather as if I knew the two greatest men there are,' she told her sister. 'AE has grown into a saint, with a head like an old Zeus – curly Greek philosopher's head, old and wise and so gentle.'[32] She visited AE during his terminal illness and attended his funeral.

Her play, *Abbé Provost*, was read by GBS, who was, she said, 'As thin as a fishing-rod and as sardonic as a knife.'[33] He thought 'it ought to do' but then forgot it. The play was a failure when staged in 1935. Her graphic picture of Mrs Shaw, bent with age, shows us Shaw at his kindest, interrupting his flow of talk 'to lift her handkerchief, or guide her cup to the little table'.[34] She thanked Joseph O'Neill for sending her his novel, *Wind from the North* (1934), based in eleventh-century Ireland. 'It made me silent with gratitude', she told him, 'when you said it was the *Scholars* that sent you back to that other world.'[35]

When Maude Clarke's doctors diagnosed inoperable cancer, it was left to Helen to tell her father. After Maude's death in November 1935, Helen's appreciation in *The Times* recalled the quality of her friend's beauty:

In her youth it had a lovely wildness, like the dancing fire of her wit, yet even then her eyes held the ancient shadows; to come upon her walking in the spring rain on the Antrim hills was to see Persephone come back from the dead, but with the knowledge of the kingdoms of it in her face.[36]

Patrick Kavanagh, on his uppers in London, appealed to Helen. She welcomed him like a prodigal son and gave him money. She urged him to write *The Green Fool* and, as he said, 'introduced me to the Promised Land'.[37]

When Paul Henry's autobiography was published, she wrote to him to praise it: 'And now I have this glorious book – it is not fair that anyone should paint and write so superbly.'[38] He had held an exhibition in Oxford soon after Helen's arrival but the *cognoscenti* preferred etchings of old masters to original Irish landscapes and he sold only one picture. He invited Helen to tea and gave her 'Early Morning in Connemara', a recent painting marked £50. 'I'd far rather you had it', he said, 'than sell it to somebody who wouldn't like it the way you do.'

'Do you remember a white hawthorn against a valley you were once going to paint –', she asked him, comparing in her mind his art and the translator's. 'You told me about it, and the ivory was just going yellow, and you went back to get it down before it would fall. Did you ever make a picture of it, or is it one of the things you'll have forever because you *didn't* paint it?'[39]

On learning from William Rothenstein, the painter, that his former teacher Alphonse Legros, when poor and unknown, had been 'discovered' by Baudelaire and that Legros put Swinburne in touch with Baudelaire, Helen insisted that he must pass this knowledge on to Enid Starkie. The latter had not yet evolved into the legendary party-goer at Oxford, conspicuous in her favoured scarlet and blue. Helen's first impression, indeed, of the Dublin girl, a student of nineteenth-century French literature, had been of a 'terribly shy little animal' that would run off if she lifted her hand or spoke too quickly. Enid valued Helen Waddell's judgment and submitted typescripts to her for constructive criticism. When Constable rejected Miss Starkie's *Baudelaire*, Helen disagreed with the verdict and drafted a letter to Victor Gollancz, who accepted it at once.

'You haven't mastered the English balance and the English rhythm,'[40] Helen told her on another occasion but she was moved

in 1938 when she read the typescript of Enid's *Arthur Rimbaud*.
'Once or twice I've suggested lowering the intensity a little . . .
Again I've cut the adverbs now and then . . . the nearer the bone
the better the prose.' But she tempered her criticism graciously,
'It is my own eternal struggle to combine feeling and austerity of
expression.'[41]

In 'Seisin', a short story written in 1915, she described the Great
War as a conflict over clear-cut issues – 'a war, in fact, where one
had regimental bands; not the strange old surging whirlpool of
sentiment and memory and bitterness that stirs in every Ulster
twilight when a sorry little flute plays "The Boyne Water" over
the darkening fields'.[42]

Helen would have liked to 'bury Irish politics in the Red Sea'
but her eighteenth-century kinsman, James Porter, was hanged
before the door of his manse in 1798, her father had favoured
Home Rule and in the Belfast of her twenties she had regarded
Sir Edward Carson as a sinister figure. 'I know the old kindly
tolerance, and I saw it stiffen – under his hand – into obstinacy
and hate.'[43]

Her sympathy went instinctively to the losing side – 'Just as
my head was with the Roundheads, and my heart distinctly
Royalist.' Politics dejected her but could not be avoided. 'One
can be a Home Ruler, and loyal to the greater issue as well.
Witness the Redmonds and Professor T.M. Kettle, and hundreds
of less-known Irishmen.'[44]

Six Belfast youths were sentenced to death by hanging in
August 1942 for the murder of a policeman. The House of
Commons was not in session and the Attorney-General of
Northern Ireland refused to grant an appeal to the House of
Lords. 'Is his case then so weak that it is unable to support the
journey to Westminster?' Helen Waddell asked in a letter of pro-
test to *The Times* that may have helped to gain a reprieve from
capital punishment.[45]

IV

When George Saintsbury, her friend of twenty years, died in
1933, Helen's note of appreciation recalled him 'in the Augustan
twilight of the house of his last inhabiting, a solitary indomitable

figure with straggling grey hair and black skull-cap, gaunt as
Merlin and islanded in a fast-encroaching sea of books . . . '. He
had directed that no biography should be written:

the refusal, in an age crazed for personal publicity, is a gesture so characteristic
of him that it uplifts the heart. This is the man we knew: not the Johnsonian
Saintsbury who loved to fold his legs and have his talk out: not the Meredi-
thian Saintsbury, emerging from his cellar with a bearded Hermitage reverently
and triumphantly bestowed: but the solitary scholar who was his own best
company . . . reading, reading, reading through the small hours in the familiar
chair with the two tall candlesticks behind it. And their light falls, not on his
face, but on the open book.[46]

Miss Waddell collected a sufficiency of honorary degrees,
including the D.Litt. of Columbia University. New York City
fascinated her, its skyscrapers worthy of Lucifer and its great
hospitals exemplifying Christian compassion.

> Lucifer, once the Light-bringer.
> Yet even in darkness
> Thou hast builded a house of light,
> By the East River
> A House for the sick and the dying, that sits like God
> With His stark head of truth, and mercy on His great knees.[47]

She remained in London during the war and edited *Nineteenth
Century and After*. When the Luftwaffe first broke through the
city's defences and left it burning, she turned to the second book
of the *Aeneid*: 'Come is the ending day, Troy's hour is come, /
The ineluctable hour.' She was consoled by Virgil's lines, knowing
that the destruction of Troy was a prelude to greater glory.[48]

For most of her adult life, Helen was prone to periods of
fatigue with occasional 'collapses'. Wartime stiffened her morale
and victory was expected to be accompanied by a salutary
resurgence of energy. The immediate post-war years, however,
were marred for Helen by the worry of her nephew's illness
(tuberculosis) and her brother-in-law's decline – the Rev. J.D.
Martin died on 5 December 1946. She was pleased, nevertheless,
to be invited to deliver the eighth W.P. Ker Memorial Lecture
at Glasgow on 28 October 1947, having yet no reason to view it
as a testing challenge.

'I've been a very dead dog since collapse on Easter Sunday but
cheerfuller every day . . . ', she told her sister, rambling on opti-

mistically about a projected translation of the *Aeneid*.[49] She also
planned to work at the British Museum on a biography of John
of Salisbury, an amplification of the earlier essay:

it was at Chartres that John of Salisbury came, in the phrase of his beloved
Petronius, to the harbour of a stilled desire. Thirty years before he had come
there to read 'the heathen writers, with whom is bound up the life of human
learning', and though Bernard's humanism was already gone from the schools,
the 'divine idea' had taken a shrine, not

> Of crystal flesh wherein to shine

but of living stone. The West Portal of the Cathedral had even then been
building; in these last decades of the century it stood, a new and gracious miracle.
Dead kings and queens, the familiar faces of Donatus and Plato and Aristotle
looked down upon him, and through the blue of the western lancets he saw
the light, as he had once seen it through a sapphire, 'become a purer heaven'.[50]

Her lecture in Glasgow, 'Poetry in the Dark Ages', a spell-
binding performance, was to be her last appearance on a rostrum.
She now sensed that her well-being was threatened by nature's
insidious and malign attack. She felt in a 'fog', lacking creativity
and affected by 'what the Desert Fathers called *accidia*, a kind of
melancholy that paralysed the soul' and she was frightened by
it.[51] Fissures in her memory broadened insidiously; her speed of
recall was slower, her powers of association retarded – but the
doctors attributed it reassuringly to anaemia.

She corrected the proofs of her *Stories from Holy Writ*, which
was published in 1949, and her tribute to Stephen Gwynn appeared
in *The Times* on 19 June 1950. The Irish writer's aggregate
qualities and his 'European mind' made her think of the Blessed
Alcuin: 'at bedrock level, Alcuin was a man of York, sprung
from the field and rock above Spurn Head, and Gwynn a son of
the O'Briens and of a rectory in Donegal. It was Charlemagne
who called Alcuin "Horace", and it might well have been Stephen's
middle name; but the iron that was in Horace as well as the
amenity was in those two also.'

Organic dementia, though relentlessly progressive, is generally
slow to declare itself in its true colours. According to Dame
Felicitas Corrigan, her biographer, Helen was 'fully and painfully
aware of the gradual failure of her mental powers', yet able to
joke about it at first, recalling wryly the words of a schoolfriend
to a teacher in Japan: '*O Masa san*, my intelligence is not work-

ing.'[52] Her doctors evidently concealed their suspicions and in the absence of firm direction she decided to buy a bottle of Metatone or Ferrsolate and forget the medical profession.

By the early 1950s she had been sent unavailingly to medical consultants and her personality change was apparent to relatives and concerned friends. Her tribute in *The Times* (a translation of a ninth-century lament for a dead abbess) to Elizabeth Lucas, a friend who died on 11 December 1951, was pathetically apt though completed some years earlier:

Thou hast come safe to port,
I still at sea,
The light is on thy head,
Darkness in me . . . [53]

A friend from Paris, visiting in 1952, found Helen sitting before a picture of Christ stumbling under the cross. 'My cross is heavy too and is crushing me,' she said with tears in her eyes. 'But looking at Him I try to carry it without being too complaining and sorry for myself.'[54]

With some assistance she managed to make a recording for the BBC in 1955; but the struggling letters quoted in her biography confirm her plight: 'Darling, would there be any chance of seeing you – I have a half-dream that you came. But when it's warmer – I wonder if my darlings will get over the water abroad. My dears, will you say your prayers for me, for I sure did very little as regards the Parable of the Talents.'[55]

By 1957, to judge from entries in her sister's diary, her behaviour when visiting Kilmacrew was that of a fully demented person. 'Helen had a bath at 4 a.m. and demanded her breakfast.' 'Helen disappeared – Billy found her wandering in the bog.' 'Helen extremely cross . . . Helen is collapsed – back to childhood – even worse. God help me to keep cheery and bright . . . '.[56]

When her dearest friend, the elderly Otto Kyllman, died in May 1959 – he had lived in her house for several years in a platonic relationship – she was untroubled, unaware of his passing. Her nephew, Dr Mayne Waddell of Glossop, and her friend Brice Clarke advised on her custody. She would hardly settle at Kilmacrew but might stay contentedly in London in the home of her former housekeeper, Mrs Luff, who lived in Camden Town. Fortunately, this plan worked.

For all that present knowledge can tell, Alzheimer's disease appears to be a merciless penalty gratuitously imposed by nature.[57] It destroys the grey matter of the brain, where an accumulation of silver-staining plaques and fibrillary tangles replaces the deeply layered nerve cells. After a period of bewildered confusion, the last vestiges of intellect disappear and uncomprehending relatives are left to cope with the appalling consequence. 'What has brought her to this?' her puzzled sister asked, 'A fate so uncalled-for.' Her nephew, Dr Waddell, felt angry, linking Helen's ill-health to the war. Characteristically, their reactions expressed the need to understand and the sense of outrage and loss at the pitiable and unacceptable transformation.

Only a mystic can see gain in such a situation but Helen's biographer, a Benedictine nun, pictured her, 'Mute, unheeding, unfeeling, blind to all beauty, a stranger to the family she had so loved . . . ' and, pondering the triune nature of man, body, soul and spirit, asked undespairingly: 'What mighty work was being wrought in and by her spirit?'[58] This trustful sublimation of sorrow would have appealed in her prime to Helen, herself a mystic, remembering the fortitude of Boethius who, within his dungeon in Pavia, saw 'not so much infinite darkness, as a multitude of quiet stars'.[59]

Her confusion and disorientations gave way to a state of gentle mindlessness in which she existed in Camden Town until her death from pneumonia on 5 March 1965 in a hospital on Highgate Hill, named for Dick Whittington. She died in spring – not, as she had predicted, in the desolation of the year:

> I think it will be winter when I die,
> For no one from the North could die in Spring –
> And so the heather will be green and grey;
> And the bog-cotton will have blown away,
> And there will be no yellow on the whin.[60]

She was buried a few days later with her ancestors in the churchyard of Magherally, a few miles from Kilmacrew House.

The Irish dimension is represented in the posthumously published *More Latin Lyrics* by St Columbanus ('O mortal life, naught but a road, a fleeting ghost, an emptiness, a cloud uncertain and frail, a shadow and a dream')[61] and by an unidentified poet, 'Hibernicus Exul at the court of Charlemagne: Jonathan Swift at the court of St James'. Charlemagne was succeeded by Louis the Pious, a king who rarely smiled: 'In his reign the Church begins to bear hard on the wandering Irishmen.'[62]

This book, edited by Dame Felicitas Corrigan (1977), was reviewed by Peter Dronke (the present professor of medieval Latin at Cambridge University), who attributed Miss Waddell's record of success 'to her being unafraid, in her writing, of expressing her own imaginative warmth: she both perceived the ardent emotions that were at play in the realm she studied and coloured that realm with ardent emotions of her own'.[63] He recognized her genius for discovering 'moments of rare poetry in the midst of long tracts of pedestrian verse' but scolded her for using archaisms ('"yea" and "yon", "ne'er" and "o'er"') in her translations. More recently and briefly, David Parlett (1986) has referred to *The Wandering Scholars* as being 'long on style and enthusiasm, short on texts and specifics, but with many valuable references and observations'.[64]

In his penetrating review, Peter Dronke remarked that 'for all its verve' *Peter Abelard* cannot 'match the original letters of the two lovers in their rich diversity of thought and feeling and their complete freedom from sentimentality and coyness'. But who would expect it to do so? Enough that the celebrated love-story remains in print and has reappeared in many languages. He detected 'serious gaps' in her representation of medieval Latin poetry and complained that the choice for her *Mediaeval Latin Lyrics*, with its emphasis on 'wine, women and song' during the period from the tenth to the thirteenth centuries, 'might well suggest to non-specialists an operetta world rather than the immense range of Latin poetic art at this time . . . '. He accused her of 'a certain lack of intellectual rigour' in the selection of original texts.[65]

Could she have read his charges she would have had a sense of *déjà vu*. She had long ago denied an apparent preference for 'the hilarity and mockery of the last masks of paganism . . . to the *sanctum saeculare* of the mediaeval hymns'.[66] She had already explained with disarming honesty her seemingly unaccountable omissions – 'I tried to translate them and could not.'[67] As for 'intellectual rigour' – unlike physical rigour it cannot be measured

with a stopwatch on the running-track. But she had stood up to
G.C. Coulton and routed him, and Dronke himself had supported her against Otto Schumann in her intuitive earlier dating
of the *Carmina Burana*. And besides, during the period in
question when *Adoro te devote*, the focus of Dronke's complaint,
was translated, she had endured rumours of war, the blitz and
finally the early inroads of a progressive malady. Tolerant of older
scholars, as likely as not she would have accepted criticism from a
younger voice with equanimity. But she had supped with Saintsbury and who could blame her had she bridled?

Dronke's more positive evaluations welcomed 'many of the
finest translations she ever did' in the volume under review,
reserving special praise for those from Petronius and Boethius; he
compared Helen's achievement with that of Wolfram von den
Steinen, discussed the source and dating of certain unidentified
pieces and placed her rendering of *Pie Pelicane, Iesu Domine* . . .
beside Crashaw's superior rendering. These highly specialized
issues, vastly interesting though they may be, are beyond the
judgment of the common reader, who will probably feel more at
ease with William Doolin's pencilled notes of appreciation recently
discovered in the surgeon-editor's copy of *The Wandering Scholars*
purchased from a second-hand bookseller.[68]

Doolin, perhaps recalling his own *Wanderjahr*, relished her pictures of Irishmen 'determined to "walk the world"' and enjoyed
her stories of their adventures. Sitting with his patron over the
wine, Johannes Scottus Eriugena was asked: 'What is there between
sottum et Scottum?' and replied, 'The breadth of the table, Sire.'[69]
Another Irish scholar, begging the loan of a book, offered the *De
Musica* of Boethius as pledge and called the abbot 'flower and
paradox of the holy church of God'. 'I cannot live in such poverty', yet another complains, 'having naught to eat or drink save
exceeding bad bread and the least particle of abominable beer.'[70]

Some have fled the Vikings only to find 'the terrible beaked
prows appear in the Meuse'. Everywhere manuscripts are destroyed. 'Hucbald of St Amand, sitting down to write his history,
laments the loss of all his materials, just as historians lament the
blowing up of the Four Courts in Dublin.'[71]

Doolin approved of the decree of Giraldus Cambrensis that
'the man of letters sits in his chimney corner with a book, and is

his own best company';[72] he smiled at Helen Waddell's recognition of 'dilutior' as an incomparable word for a relaxed state of incipient inebriation.[73] He was pleased to have her as guide in Pavia, a place honoured in medical history, and as a teacher in St Vincent's Hospital he understood how John of Salisbury found teaching 'a quickening of his own studies'.[74] It amused him to read that 'Alcuin, waking at night and watching the devils nip the toes of the other monks in the dormitory, called anxiously to mind that he had scamped the Psalms to read the Aeneid.'[75] He noted that the twelfth-century injunction forbidding monks and canons regular to read either medicine or civil law caused defections, and was charmed by lines from the *Carmina Burana* – 'O tender laughter of those wanton lips / That draw all eyes upon them . . . '.[76]

Helen Waddell was in her prime in 1933 when *The Wandering Scholars* was thus annotated. She survives in her books: 'The written word alone flouts destiny, / Revives the past, and gives the lie to Death.'[77]

NOTES

1. Dame Felicitas Corrigan, *Helen Waddell, A Biography* (London 1986), p. 24.
2. *Ibid.*, p. 29.
3. *Ibid.*, pp. 101–2.
4. *Ibid.*, p. 163.
5. Helen Waddell, *Lyrics from the Chinese* (London 1913), p. 33.
6. *Ibid.*, p. 8.
7. Corrigan, *op. cit.*, p. 163.
8. *Ibid.*, p. 66.
9. Monica Blackett, *The Mark of the Maker* (London 1973), p. 33.
10. Corrigan, *op. cit.*, p. 208.
11. *The Times*, 29 April 1927, p. 8.
12. Helen Waddell, 'John of Salisbury' in *Essays and Studies by Members of the English Association*, vol. 13 (Oxford 1929), pp. 28–51.
13. 'L.R.', *The Irish Statesman* (1927), 8: 476–8.
14. 'W.J.W.', *Studies* (1927), 16: 349–51.
15. Gerard Murphy, *The Irish Statesman* (1930), 10: 394–6.
16. Gerard Murphy, *The Irish Booklover* (1935), 23: 31.
17. T.B. Rudmose-Brown, *Dublin Magazine* (1934), NS vol. ix: 1, 71–2; Helen Waddell, *ibid.*, 2, 79–82; Rudmose-Brown, 3, 90–2.
18. Padraic Colum: typescript in J.S. Starkey papers, NLI, MS. 15,567.
19. Helen Waddell, *The Desert Fathers* (London 1987), *passim*.
20. 'Colm', *The Irish Booklover* (1935), 23: 79.

21. Helen Waddell, *More Latin Lyrics* (ed. Dame Felicitas Corrigan) (London 1976), p. 375.
22. Helen Waddell, *The Wandering Scholars* (London 1987), p. 38.
23. *Ibid.*, p. 53.
24. TCD MS. 4633/809 a.
25. TCD MS. 4633/815.
26. Helen Waddell's introduction to W.F. Marshall's *Ballads and Verses from Tyrone* (Dublin 1929), pp. 9–12.
27. Monica Blackett, *op. cit.*, p. 100.
28. *Ibid.*, p. 221.
29. *Ibid.*, p. 107.
30. *Ibid.*, p. 115.
31. *Ibid.*, p. 117.
32. *Ibid.*, p. 118.
33. *Ibid.*, p. 119.
34. *Ibid.*, p. 171.
35. NLI, letter to Joseph O'Neill.
36. *The Times*, 25 November 1935; see also *Peter Abelard* (London 1950), p. 47.
37. Patrick Kavanagh, *The Green Fool* (London 1950), p. 348.
38. TCD MS. (Paul Henry papers) 314.
39. TCD, letter to Paul Henry.
40. Joanna Richardson, *Enid Starkie* (London 1973), p. 102.
41. *Ibid.*, p. 116.
42. Helen's short story, written in 1915, is published in *Irish Harvest* (ed. Robert Greacen) (Dublin 1946), pp. 144–7.
43. Corrigan, *op. cit.*, p. 182.
44. *Ibid.*, p. 184.
45. *The Times*, 28 August 1942.
46. An Appreciation by Helen Waddell in George Saintsbury, *Shakespeare* (Cambridge 1934), pp. 7–14.
47. *More Latin Lyrics*, p. 380.
48. Helen Waddell, *Poetry in the Dark Ages* (London 1948).
49. Corrigan, *op. cit.*, p. 344.
50. Helen Waddell, 'John of Salisbury', p. 49.
51. Corrigan, *op. cit.*, p. 336.
52. *Ibid.*, p. 350.
53. *Ibid.*, p. 317.
54. Blackett, *op. cit.*, p. 188.
55. Corrigan, *op. cit.*, p. 353.
56. *Ibid.*, p. 355.
57. Alois Alzheimer (1864–1915) was born in Marktbreit-am-Main, the son of a lawyer. He studied medicine in Berlin, Würzburg and Tübingen and held posts in Heidelberg, Munich and Breslau. He practised psychiatry and was attracted to the study of changes in the brain associated with certain mental disorders. At a meeting of the South West German Society of Alienists in Tübingen in the first week of November 1906 he described

the post-mortem findings in a 51-year-old married woman who had been severely demented for five years before her death. The brain was atrophied and he demonstrated a clumping and distortion of the cortical neurofibrils which is now associated with his name.

58. Corrigan, *op. cit.*, p. 356.
59. *The Wandering Scholars*, p. xxix.
60. *More Latin Lyrics*, p. 375.
61. *Ibid.*, p. 214.
62. *Ibid.*, p. 214.
63. Peter Dronke, 'The Medieval Voice', *Times Literary Supplement*, 17 June 1977, 727.
64. David Parlett, *Selection from the Carmina Burana* (Harmondsworth 1986), p. 255.
65. His most specific charge was that she used the traditional *Adoro te devote, latens Deitas / Quae sub his figuris vere latitas* . . . despite the availability since 1929 of the correct version taken from the earliest manuscripts by Dom André Wilmart: *Adoro devote, latens veritas, / te qui sub his formis vere latitas* . . . Did Miss Waddell overlook Wilmart's work or did she ignore it to favour the familiar and established version?
66. Helen Waddell, *Mediaeval Latin Lyrics* (Harmondsworth 1952), Note to the 4th ed., p. 10.
67. *Ibid.*, p. 8.
68. MS. RCSI.
69. *The Wandering Scholars*, 6th ed. (London 1932), p. 52.
70. *Ibid.*, p. 59.
71. *Ibid.*, p. 63.
72. *Ibid.*, p. 113.
73. *Ibid.*, pp. 7–8.
74. *Ibid.*, p. 172.
75. *Ibid.*, p. xxiii.
76. *Ibid.*, p. 117.
77. From 'To Eigilus, on the book that he had written' by Hrabanus Maurus in *Mediaeval Latin Lyrics*, p. 119.

11

Portraits of Alcoholism by James Joyce and Malcolm Lowry

JAMES Joyce and Malcolm Lowry were separated in their incarnations by the Irish Sea and twenty-seven years. According to the younger man, they met in Paris, a chance encounter in the Luxembourg Gardens where he found Joyce smiling and approachable.[1] But Malcolm's fictions tended to displace facts in conversation and the discussion with Joyce may have been wholly imaginary. One could, however, draw up a list of parallels in their lives: eye afflictions; letters to an intellectual patron, Ibsen / Conrad Aiken; love of music, bel canto and opera / jazz; cinema – Joyce organized the Volta Cinema / Lowry a film-buff. Both learned Norwegian; Lowry had psychiatric treatment, Joyce's friends thought he'd benefit from it; Lowry sailed from New York to Genoa in the SS *Giacoma*; the Dollarton shack and 7 Eccles Street were ravaged by builders.

Unimportant parallels in their writings may also be adduced: the *Rosevan* with bricks from Bridgwater in *Ulysses*, the ubiquitous *Oxensjerna* in *Ultramarine*; the 'Dolor! O, he dolores!' of 'Sirens' echoes in *Under the Volcano*; Granada and Gibraltar; Agenbite; impotence; 'Twinbad the bailer' in Lowry's letter to Erskine, presumably a variant of Joyce's Sinbad litany; Yvonne Constable and Gerty MacDowell are both creatures of pure pastiche.

Lowry attempted to read *Ulysses* when travelling in a train with a hangover in 1933. He must have read it on less difficult occasions but he resented suggestions from critics that he imitated Joyce. His own talents, he believed, favoured simplification of the complex whereas Joyce promoted the esoteric. Lowry admitted that he had never read *Ulysses* right through. He found it 'full of inventories' and disliked it though not necessarily because he had read sufficiently far to encounter his own name, Lowry, in a death column scanned by Leopold Bloom.

Naturally the differences in their lives and careers are more striking than my somewhat contrived list of similarities. At the Liffey-mouth, facing east, Joyce saw the black hull of the B&I boat at the North Wall. He sailed in it and followed the paths, though in a less than saintly manner, of the medieval Irish missionaries. Near Lowry's home at Caldy on the Wirral Peninsula, 'The smoke of freighters outward bound from Liverpool hung on the horizon . . .'.[2] As intrepid as Drake or the great English explorers he sought a wider world. His travels brought him to the Far East, Scandinavia, continental Europe, the United States, Mexico and Canada, where he settled – 'this strange undeserved country / whose heart is England and whose soul is Labrador'.[3]

Their fathers, brothers, wives were very different types. Joyce was a master of all styles and periods, Lowry, on the whole, less accomplished – 'the desire to write is a disease like any other disease; and what one writes if one is to be any good, must be rooted firmly in some sort of autochthony. And there I abdicate. I can no more create than fly.'[4]

They are drawn together, finally, as authors of two of the great novels of the twentieth century, *Ulysses* and *Under the Volcano*.

Alcoholism is the most prevalent disease in *Dubliners* and examples are readily cited: Tom Kernan ('Grace'), Mrs Sinico ('A Painful Case'), Farrington ('Counterparts'); they are presented as miscreants or, with the exception of Freddy Malins, as joyless victims.[5] *A Portrait*'s texture is different. Stephen Dedalus has not yet experienced the delusive pleasures and *camaraderie* of the taverns but even as a tiny boy he is aware of adult rituals, the great stone jar of whiskey, the decanter and the glass which his father offers to a Christmas guest – 'a thimbleful, John, he said, just to whet your appetite'.[6]

A paradox attaching to wine puzzles the little lad; though nasty to smell it had a lovely name, evocative of sunshine and white houses.[7] How could the erring Clongownians have drunk the altar wine? The sacristy was a holy place, the wine sacramental.

Stephen, in adolescence, listens to his father's monologue in the train, 'a tale broken by sighs or draughts from his pocket-flask . . .'.[8] At breakfast next morning he attempts to distract attention from his parent's giveaway tremor and later in the day is a cold observer of his father's Cork cronies who toast the past.

On another occasion he can't control his impatience as he paces to and fro between Clontarf chapel and Byron's public house where Simon Dedalus is installed with Dan Crosby, the tutor. His father, he tells Cranly, is 'a drinker, a good fellow . . . ' and his friend is amused to think that such a man chose to work in a distillery.[9]

Stephen bows to other desires ('Girls demure and romping. All fair or auburn . . .),[10] engages in other conflicts and passes judgment on his father's way of life. Alcoholism is portrayed indirectly through his disapproval. Not for him, just yet, the cordiality of Dublin's hostelries so well represented by Oliver Gogarty in 'The Hay Hotel':

> There is a window stuffed with hay
> Like herbage in an oven cast;
> And there we came at break of day
> To soothe ourselves with light repast:
> And men who worked before the mast
> And drunken girls delectable:
> A future symbol of our past
> You'll, maybe, find the Hay Hotel.[11]

Dana Hilliot, Lowry's surrogate in *Ultramarine*, has a more abrupt initiation to bacchanalian rites in a string of dockside bars between Liverpool and the Far East. His mature equivalent, Bill Plantagenet, moves with a certain inevitability towards the psychiatric ward at Bellevue Hospital in Lowry's Hemingwayesque introductory paragraphs to *Lunar Caustic*.

Faced with the realities of a mariner's life, Hilliot realizes that he 'is a man who believed himself to live in inverted, or introverted commas' but resents Andy, the cook, calling him 'just a bloody twat – '. 'You're one of the most regular booze artists I ever struck,' another shipmate tells him while a third recalled an occasion when young Hilliot was 'so drunk that he tried to wrap the deck around him for a blanket'.[12]

When Plantagenet / Lowry is interviewed by Dr Claggart, an overworked Bellevue psychiatrist, he wonders (anticipating the late Dr R.D. Laing) if the doctor ever asked himself what point there was in adjusting poor lunatics to a mischievous world over which merely more subtle lunatics exerted almost supreme hegemony, where neurotic behaviour was the rule, and there was nothing but hypocrisy to answer the flames of evil . . .[13]

Dubliners and the *Portrait* may be placed in parallel with *Ultramarine* and *Lunar Caustic*, the apprentice texts with which Joyce and Lowry perfected their craft before venturing to fashion the elaborate magnificence of *Ulysses* and *Under the Volcano*, their encyclopedic and cabbalistic masterpieces. Stuart Gilbert, to mention just one exegesist, has tabulated the organs, art, colour, etc. of Joyce's symbol-laden episodes.[14] Lowry himself, in the celebrated letter to Jonathan Cape, explained that the Consul's folly images 'the universal drunkenness of mankind during the war'.[15] Avoiding this complex web which affords unlimited scope for conjecture and gives licence to the more imaginative critics I shall follow the sufficiently complex theme of alcoholism as portrayed in the major novels. *Wonders are many* . . . Lowry reminds us, quoting Sophocles, *and none is more wonderful than man.* His vices, Lowry might have added, are not the least part of that wonder.

Neither author adds to our knowledge of the aetiology of alcoholism, a disorder of multi-factorial origin, but their expertise and dearly bought experience enabled them to supply a variety of inimitable 'clinical pictures' of alcohol abusers, the striking difference in their dark and lively frescoes being that Joyce's sharply drawn examples are objective and pejorative, Lowry's subjective and sympathetic. In the letter already referred to he admits to Cape that his talent as an author 'is subjective rather than objective, a better equipment, in short, for a certain kind of poet than novelist'.[16] Lowry's verses actually take drink and inebriates as frequent themes, matters which would be alien to Joyce's delicate lyrics. The love of family shines from poems such as 'On the Beach at Fontana' and 'Ecce Puer'. A broader charity, albeit bizarre and self-interested, inspired the following lines by Lowry:

> God give those drunkards drink who wake at dawn
> Gibbering on Beelzebub's bosom, all outworn,
> As once more through the windows they espy
> Looming, the dreadful Pontefract of day.[17]

Lowry's letters make no attempt to soften his vicissitudes. 'This is not the cry of the boy who cried wolf,' he assured the critic John Davenport. 'It is the wolf itself that cries for help.'[18] Joyce's letters (other than private effusions for Nora) were usually models of discretion radiating good-humoured acceptance of his trying eye complaint.

The drinkers in *Ulysses* include the students whose philosophy is *carpe diem* – they drink all they can whenever they can get it; the soldiers, salesmen and newspapermen for whom alcohol is an occupational risk; the chronic soaks such as Simon Dedalus who still retain a measure of social acceptability, unlike Bob Doran, a psychopathic drunkard who on 16 June 1904 was 'on one of his periodic bends'; the respectable regulars such as Mr Power and his friends who favour James Kavanagh's wine-rooms.

Moderate in all things, Leopold Bloom takes one glass of burgundy: '– God Almighty couldn't make him drunk, Nosey Flynn said firmly. Slips off when the fun gets too hot.'[19] Paddy Leonard is offended when his 'alemates', Tom Rochford and Bantam Lyons, ask for water and stone ginger. 'Two fellows that would suck whisky off a sore leg.'[20] Molly Bloom fancies rich, coloured liqueurs and occasionally drinks port. She recalls Tom Kernan and the late Paddy Dignam 'always stuck up in some pub corner'. She is puzzled by the students' abandon – 'what do they find to gabber about all night squandering money and getting drunker and drunker couldn't they drink water'.[21]

Buck Mulligan, the archetypal student, is thrilled by the prospect of an influx of funds – 'Four shining sovereigns . . . We'll have a glorious drunk to astonish the druidy druids'[22] and student revels are depicted in Holles Street and Nighttown where 'reserved young Stephen, he was the most drunken that demanded still of more mead'.[23] Bloom finally links him to the cabmen's shelter, where they encounter Corley, whose breath is 'redolent of rotten cornjuice',[24] and see the red-bearded sailor, whose eyes are 'bunged up from excessive use of booze . . .'.[25]

Tom Kernan enjoys a thimbleful of gin that warms his vitals. A snappy dresser and self-satisfied man-about-town, he is unaware that Molly Bloom remembers him as 'that drunken little barrelly man that bit his tongue off falling down the mens WC drunk in some place or other . . .'.[26]

Leopold Bloom thinks of Martin Cunningham: 'And that awful drunkard of a wife of his . . .'.[27] He approves of the anti-treating league and regards drink as the curse of Ireland. 'Lord Iveagh once changed a seven-figure cheque for a million in the bank of Ireland. Shows you the money to be made out of porter.'[28]

The indictment of alcohol in *Under the Volcano* is equally un-equivocal but the fuller exploration of the mind of an individual addict, Geoffrey Firmin, ex-British consul in Quauhnahuac, introduces an element of ambivalence. The Mexican background is brilliantly described and additional characters are introduced, attractive and grotesque. Outstanding among the former is Dr Arturo Vigil, *Medico Cirujano y Partero*, who speaks in imperfect English to Monsieur Laruelle of the Consul's alcoholic excesses. 'Sickness is not only in body, but in that part used to be call: soul. Poor your friend he spend his money on earth in such continuous tragedies.'[29] Vigil's own partiality for *anis* causes in him a conflict of conscience – 'for we doctors must comport ourselves like apostles'.[30]

The Consul, Malcolm Lowry's surrogate, drinks beer, whiskey, tequila and mescal (bay rum if the impulse takes him) and his unhappy plight is steadily revealed. A flashback introduces him to us indirectly as Vigil and Jacques Laruelle (Yvonne's lover) recall the awful events a year earlier on the Day of the Dead when the Consul's half-brother, Hugh Firmin (who, too, has succumbed to Yvonne's charms), is the only survivor of the little party that set out for the Farolito, a pub in Parian under the volcano. Mistaken for a spy, the Consul is shot and tipped into the *barranca*. Yvonne is killed by a runaway horse, a mysterious creature that has crossed their paths several times that day. (Jan Gabrial, Lowry's first wife, thought it 'an interesting quirk' that she was killed by a stallion, an unintended Freudian overtone.)[31]

We meet him in person, sockless because of alcoholic neuritis, on that actual Day of the Dead when Yvonne, his divorced wife, attempts to return to him. He has the shakes, 'the rajah shakes' and incipient DTs, which he hopes to cure with mescal – 'the drink that I can never believe even in raising to my lips is real . . .'. He is mocked in the street – 'You-are-a-man-who-like-much-Vine' – and humiliated in different ways that leave him fit com-panion only for the pariahs.[32]

Lowry's surrogate is a past master of evasion and subterfuge retaining insight enough to sense his doom but asserting a sacramental dedication to alcohol. Who but the addict understands the fervour of his own enthraldom: 'What beauty can compare to that of a cantina in the early morning?' [33] The Consul knows, better than others, that he is 'like a great explorer who has discovered some extraordinary land from which he can never return to give his knowledge of the world: but the name of this land is hell'.[34]

Under the Volcano portrays the loss that is the alcoholic's lot, the estrangement of friends and lovers, and underlines, without explaining, the inebriate's expectations at opening-time:

> not even the gates of heaven, opening wide to receive me, could fill me with such celestial complicated and hopeless joy as the iron screen that rolls up with a crash, as the unpadlocked jostling jalousies which admit those whose souls tremble with the drinks they carry unsteadily to their lips. All mystery, all hope, all disappointment, yes, all disaster, is here, beyond those swinging doors.[35]

This unexpected rhapsody, a paean from the addicted, has no counterpart in *Ulysses* unless concealed somewhere in the phantasmagoria of the Circe episode,[36] and when Joyce's and Lowry's contrasting attitudes are considered, the latter's 'innocence' supplies an explanation. Joyce grew up in the ambience of alcohol and learned subconsciously to loathe it. Attracted, nevertheless, at a personal level by the hereditary factor he was obliged to moderate his drinking by nagging relatives. Lowry, raised in an abstemious English household, embarked with unpredictable vigour and with no natural immunity on a fresh adventure. He was soon rejected by his staid family as a disgrace and disappointment but to no avail. Believing in a 'Brotherhood of Alcohol', Lowry never quite out-grew his fixation on bohemianism. Donald Newlove's survey of alcoholic writers, *Those Drinking Days*, found him unique among the topers, convinced that 'his genius sprang from drink'.[37] The insight which allowed Joyce to describe himself as 'a man of small virtue inclined to alcoholism' separates him prognostically from Lowry, an uncompromising figure who argued with Dr Raymond and refused to believe that for him there was no middle road of moderation. Joyce had the additional protection of a more cohesive family structure than Lowry's.[38] The latter, a 'remittance man', was tolerated at a distance (a 'bloody nuisance!')[39]

while Margerie Bonner, his second wife, was an indulgent keeper.[40]
The measure of their drinking habits also differed and Lowry's
was gargantuan –

> The only hope is the next drink.
> If you like, you take a walk.
> No time to stop and think,
> The only hope is the next drink
> Useless trembling on the brink . . . [41]

'*That dreadful man Mr Joyce*', wrote 'Chanel' in *St Stephen's*
(1901) 'is quite a respectable person in private life.'[42] By 1904
when he ran off with Nora Barnacle, a chambermaid from Finn's
Hotel, the aura of respectability was forfeited. An initial affectation
for sack, the tipple of the Elizabethan poets, was replaced by a
taste for Guinness's less expensive porter and Gogarty's limerick
celebrates the transformation:

> There is a young fellow named Joyce
> Who possesseth a sweet tenor voice.
> He goes to the Kips
> With a psalm on his lips
> And biddeth the harlots rejoice. [43]

Stanislaus Joyce believed that Gogarty urged his brother to drink
in order 'to break his spirit'.[44] This is unlikely and when Stannie
arrived in Trieste he exerted himself to curb the elder brother's
natural waywardness. Liberated from this restraint Joyce kicked
over the traces in Rome, where he fell into bad company and
was robbed of his wages on the night before he left the city. In
Paris Hemingway regarded him as a 'rummy' and Robert
McAlmon, the author of *Being Geniuses Together*, learned that if
Joyce recited Dante in a café he would stay out till morning. But
Nora voiced her disapproval and disciplined him in a way that
Margerie never managed to do with Lowry.

Advancing years, literary acclaim and family responsibilities
altered Joyce. A close friend, Louis Gillet, recalled that when
they met in the late afternoons Joyce would sit down, sigh, and
order lime-blossom or vervain tea. The French academician's
impression that Joyce did not drink was not correct but he
succeeded in controlling the habit.[45]

The youngest son of a well-to-do Lancashire cotton-broker,
Lowry went to sea in a ship of the Blue Funnel line at seventeen,

took a third-class degree at Cambridge and augmented his education in Soho, where snorters of whiskey before breakfast and treble gins to cure hangovers distinguished him in the Fitzroy Tavern as a redoubtable drinker.[46]

While holidaying in Granada in 1933, he fell for an attractive New Yorker, Jan Gabrial. They wed in Paris on 6 January 1934 but the marriage was unstable and when she left him after a few months he followed her to New York. Infernal aspects of Manhattan registered on his sensibility – 'the whole mechanic calamity of the rocking city, with the screaming of suicides, of girls tortured in hotels for transients'[47] – and his drinking led to his voluntary admission to Bellevue Hospital.

Lowry and Jan patched up their marriage. She accompanied him to Hollywood and Mexico. They arrived in Acapulco on the Day of the Dead and went on to Cuernavaca in the Sierra Madre, where, in a rented villa, Lowry worked on the first version of *Under the Volcano*. Cuernavaca offered a beautiful landscape and a tempting variety of new drinks, including pulque, tequila and mescal. Binges alternated with sober intervals but the arrival of visitors such as Conrad Aiken or Arthur and Ara Calder-Marshall led to intensified sprees. When Jan finally left him he abandoned any pretence at control and sank through a series of disreputable cantinas to spend Christmas 1937 in the lock-up. 'Have now [he wrote to Aiken] reached condition of amnesia, breakdown, heartbreak and consumption, cholera, alcoholic poisoning and God will not like to know what else, if he has to, which is damned doubtful.' [48]

It is unlikely that Lowry was actually deported from Mexico. His father's lawyers persuaded him to leave in September 1938 and arranged transport to Los Angeles. He looked up Jan, who when she saw him 'very drunk and very boisterous' dissolved into tears.[49] Reconcilement was improbable but she urged Malcolm's father to have him sent to the Menninger Clinic; instead he was 'dried out' in the more spartan surroundings of La Crescenta. Jan and Malcolm were drifting apart and she divorced him when she learned that he was involved with another woman. This was Margerie Bonner, a starlet of the silent films, whom he married when his divorce came through, having lived with her meanwhile in British Columbia.

It was Lowry's lawyer who selected Vancouver as his next place of residence, for when he realized that Jan's plea for divorce charged his client with lack of support, extreme cruelty and habitual intoxication, he decided to get him across the border. Lowry made one attempt to visit Margerie but was turned back incapably drunk at Blaine, Washington. Margerie then gave up her job and joined him in Canada.

His discontent in Vancouver evoked a sonnet:

> I hope, although I doubt it, God knows
> This place where chancres blossom like the rose,
> For on each face is such a hard despair
> That nothing like a grief could enter there.
> And on this scene from all excuse exempt
> The mountains gaze in absolute contempt . . . [50]

The magnificent mountains framing the city to the north-east attracted him and at Dollarton, on the shore of Burrard Inlet and Indian Arm, he rented a fisherman's shack and later built his own timber house complete with pier. Green forest and blue sea provided a setting in which Lowry's life regained coherence. He boated, swam and chatted with the neighbours, ostensibly humble folk but actually skilled craftsmen close to nature. For long periods he drank little and his health benefited immensely.

Here he wrote *Under the Volcano* but before its acceptance for publication he unwisely returned to Mexico – 'it was like a Station of the Cross in the unfinished Oberammergau of his life' – a visit which provided material for the posthumously published *Deep as the Grave Wherein my Friend is Laid*, a curious book in which Sigbjørn Wilderness, one of Lowry's many surrogates, takes his wife, Primrose, to Mexico, the scene of his novel *The Valley of the Shadow of Death*, which features a guilt-ridden figure of authority who happens to be a consul. *Deep as the Grave* is the introspective case-book of an alcoholic writer, the confrontation by an author of his inspiration. Since Omar Khayyám nobody has looked so steadfastly into the glass as has Malcolm Lowry, who attributed to William James the statement that drinking is the poor man's symphony.

The acclaim awarded to *Under the Volcano* augmented his distress. 'Success is like some horrible disaster,' he wrote, 'Worse than your house burning . . .'. [51] The bitter recollection of the accidental burning of the Dollarton shack opened a wound. They rebuilt the house only to be threatened with eviction to facilitate local council plans. Fate expelled them like besotted innocents from the Garden of Eden.

Lowry mitigated the horror of the Consul's plight by investing him with a romantic glow and Gothic surroundings, artifices missing from Margerie's diary of actual events during their travels. Their visit to Haiti followed a predictable schedule:

> Below the Champs de Mars we go into a tiny pub only 10 ft square with a bar 2 foot long the radio plays too loudly, many Haitians come in, we drink and drink . . . They are all so clean, and happy and black and smiling – why am I afraid? Not really physically afraid but something darker and strange. Will we never leave this place? Now it is 11 and still we are here.[52]

Lowry's spree ended in the hospital, where, lacking the Consul's *brio*, he asks himself pathetically, 'Why am I always looking out of hospitals, out of windows, but especially out of hospital windows?'

They sailed from Vancouver in the *Brest*, a French cargo boat, on 7 November 1947: 'we all have benedictine in Captain's office but poor darling Malc has fantasy that he has been insulted which upsets him horribly and is not straightened out until next day . . .'. They pass through Juan de Fuca Strait (Lowry 'too excited and in an evil temper') and reach San Francisco on 11 November. 'We go to a little bar . . .', then return to the ship, where a party is in progress.

Next day – 'We have some hangover but are happy and good' – she notices storm signals in Malcolm and wonders if they should have come. But he can't stay permanently in retreat. 'Or does she deceive herself? Is the trip her own idea? She recalls Dr Rawlings ('the stinker') – '"But doctor, he needs to see people once in a while . . ." "Don't you mean that *you* need to see people?"' 'But his problem is not that of just an alcoholic or even that of a psychotic – he is a genius. God help me to understand and to help him.'

16 November: 'hangoverish and nervous. Cocktails before lunch which worries me . . .'. The pace of Malcolm's drinking increased. How could she believe in the 'new Era' he promised? She avoided a quarrel but expected the appearance of the same old rhythm – 'a few cocktails before dinner, then but a man is different, *I want to drink* after dinner – on holidays – then the aperitif before lunch and evening cocktails creeping up from 5 to

3. Now begins the signs I really dread: drinking before mirrors – the retreat into the blue lagoon, the excuses of some – any! emotional crisis, the alternate cruel and cold, shifty and calculating looks with fake affection which infuriate and sicken me.'
  23 November: 'And now we are happy! Malc the unpredictable! Oh how incredibly rich and wonderful life seems standing in the sun in the bow of the boat.'
  1 December: 'Very bad shambles at night.' The following day was their wedding anniversary.

I wake feeling so sad and despairing but trying to make vow that I will try to be gentle and good no matter what. M. looks dreadful but makes an effort and gives me lighter. I am touched and give devil his due though he has been passed out every night he has refrained from passing out in the a.m. But I am so frightened and sad, sad, and before lunch crying.

She puts on a brave face. Before lunch they drink with the Captain. *Bon anniversaire.* After lunch they buy a drink for all. Notices have been posted on their cabin door – Wedding, in Gothic letters. JUST MARRIED. *L'amour c'est l'éternel printemps.* 'We invite them all in for snorts . . .'. The party continues and Malcolm's behaviour is exemplary at dinner:

Then to room and Malcolm suddenly sort of passes out on leather seat. I have wanted love but see it is impossible and am fastidiously revolted, as so often, by his drunkenness. So I am utterly foul, hysterical and vile, smashing and horrible, we make up and go to the deck standing at rail in waning moonlight.

On 9 December Lowry lay in his bunk 'gloomy and savage' predicting death and disaster. Before dinner a thunderstorm stirred him and he rose gleefully to watch a scene that would have terrified Joyce. The English coastal lights were seen at midnight on 16 December and two days later they went ashore at Rotterdam. 'We have a delicious cherry brandy, then Malc beer and me a Bols.' They disembarked finally at Le Havre on 23 December and went on to Paris. 'We sit in a station café drinking Pernod inhaling Paris . . . excited, happy.' The Deux Magots was closed, no food served at the Flore. Finally they ate bread and ham in a bar on the rue Bonaparte and drank in 'a tiny dive', Le Tabour, which closed at midnight.

Two chaps guide us back to hotel. One is polite and charming and keeps repeatedly coming to salute: *France et Angleterre.* The other is fat and horrible

and kisses me furiously with wet fat lips. I feel utterly defiled. Row – sleep.
Morning of Xmas Eve M. wakes me, he up and dressed. I am paralysed and
cannot move.

Lowry left her at 11 a.m. on Christmas Eve and returned at 3
p.m. on Christmas Day. 'The horror of these 28 hours cannot be
told.' The arrival of his friend John Davenport, intent on a New
Year's Day binge, introduced further complications. Nevertheless
they went to Chartres next day.[53]

An episode of violence in Cassis led to Stuart Lowry being
summoned from England later in that disastrous year. Malcolm
was admitted to the American Hospital in Paris and had a further
spell in a sanatorium near Rome. Early in January 1949 he flew
to England, where he was sustained through a delay in London
airport by the company of Davenport and Calder-Marshall
before continuing the long flight to Canada fortified by alcohol
and barbiturates.

Two of Lowry's doctors, Clarence G. McNeil, a Vancouver
general practitioner, and Michael Raymond, a London psychiatrist,
have given details of their consultations. When McNeil advised
treatment for varicose veins he was struck by Lowry's depen-
dence on his wife, and his phobias – 'fear of syphilis, rashes, and
body distortion'.[54] He referred, too, to 'numerous violences',
which possibly include Lowry's fall from the pier outside the shack.
He sustained a compression fracture of the fourth dorsal vertebra
and following admission to a Catholic hospital in Vancouver was
transferred under sedation in a strait-jacket to another general
hospital. The apparitions which Lowry liked to attribute to the
religious ambience were those of delirium tremens and his story
that an exorcism was performed in the ward is hardly to be
credited.

Having consulted Sir Paul Mallinson at 50 Wimpole Street,
London, the former address of Elizabeth Barrett, Lowry was
admitted to the Atkinson Morley Hospital on 28 November
1955. In the immediate phase following his admission in a
drunken state, Michael Raymond found him objectionable and
uncooperative but soon realized Lowry's unlimited capacity for
introspective analysis. When the exhausted psychiatrist broke off
a particularly long session the patient called it 'spiritual coitus
interruptus'.[55]

The record of hospitalization in New York, Los Angeles, Vancouver and Europe would have told Dr Raymond that cure was unlikely. A measure of rehabilitation was achieved but brittle days of sobriety alternated with unrestraint until the evening of 26 June 1957, when, after the best part of a bottle of gin, Lowry swallowed possibly fifty sodium amytal capsules and died. He had remained until the end as refractory as his own Consul yet still innocently

> Weaving the vision of the unassimilable inn
> Where we may drink forever without owing
> With the door open, and the wind blowing.[56]

NOTES

1. Harvey Breit and Margerie Lowry, *Selected Letters of Malcolm Lowry* (London 1967), p. 250.
2. Malcolm Lowry, *Under the Volcano* (Harmondsworth 1977), p. 23.
3. MS. University of British Columbia, Vancouver, Lowry Collection: Box 6–25.
4. Malcolm Lowry, *Ultramarine* (Harmondsworth 1975), p. 89.
5. Discussed more fully in J.B. Lyons, *Thrust Syphilis Down to Hell* (Dublin 1988), pp. 51–9.
6. James Joyce, *A Portrait of the Artist as a Young Man* (Harmondsworth 1966), p. 28.
7. *Ibid.*, p. 47.
8. *Ibid.*, p. 87.
9. *Ibid.*, p. 241.
10. *Ibid.*, p. 251.
11. Oliver St John Gogarty, 'The Hay Hotel', *The Faber Book of Irish Verse* (ed. John Montague) (London 1974), pp. 226–7.
12. *Ultramarine*, p. 62.
13. Malcolm Lowry, *Lunar Caustic* (London 1968), p. 37.
14. Stuart Gilbert, *James Joyce's Ulysses* (Harmondsworth 1963), p. 38.
15. *Letters*, p. 66.
16. *Ibid.*, p. 59.
17. Earle Birney and Margerie Lowry (eds), *Selected Poems of Malcolm Lowry* (San Francisco 1962), p. 34.
18. *Letters*, p. 13.
19. James Joyce, *Ulysses* (Harmondsworth 1977), p. 177.
20. *Ibid.*, p. 178.
21. *Ibid.*, p. 685.
22. *Ibid.*, p. 17.
23. *Ibid.*, p. 386.
24. *Ibid.*, p. 536.

25. *Ibid.*, p. 543.
26. *Ibid.*, p. 694.
27. *Ibid.*, p. 98.
28. *Ibid.*, p. 81.
29. *Volcano*, p. 11.
30. *Ibid.*, p. 10.
31. Jan Gabrial in Gordon Bowker (ed.), *Malcolm Lowry Remembered* (London 1985), p. 209.
32. *Volcano*, p. 69.
33. *Ibid.*, p. 55.
34. *Ibid.*, p. 42.
35. *Ibid.*, p. 55.
36. Joyce told Padraic Colum (*Dublin Magazine* [1932], 7: 48) that he liked to sit at the end of the day and drink wine with friends. 'I say at the end of the day, for I would not drink wine until the sun goes down. Wine is sunshine; under the figure of wine the Creator of the Universe could manifest himself.'
37. Donald Newlove, *Those Drinking Days* (London 1981), p. 119.
38. A letter from his father in 1940 was coldly sympathetic: 'I am sorry you think you are living on the side of the moon always turned from the earth, but I didn't put you there and when you manage to turn to me, as you often do, you get help, don't you?' MS. UBC Lowry Collection 1–38.
39. Russell Lowry in Bowker, *op. cit.*, p. 165.
40. A wife's indulgence is detailed in 'Gin and Goldenrod' (*Hear Us O Lord from Heaven Thy Dwelling Place* [1969], p. 215): She has put away a bottle of gin that he has forgotten. 'Then we can have it now.' 'Sure. And we can have a cocktail when we get back.'
41. *Poems*, p. 38.
42. 'Chanel', *St Stephen's* (1901), 1: 52.
43. Stanislaus Joyce, *My Brother's Keeper* (London 1958), p. 160.
44. *Ibid.*, p. 240.
45. Richard Ellmann, *James Joyce* (London 1959), *passim*.
46. Douglas Day, *Malcolm Lowry: A Biography* (New York 1973), *passim*.
47. *Lunar Caustic*, p. 69.
48. *Letters*, p. 15.
49. Jan Gabrial in Bowker, *op. cit.*, p. 123.
50. *Poems*, p. 64.
51. *Ibid.*, p. 78.
52. MS. UBC Lowry Collection 7. 9.
53. Details of the European visit are given in Margerie's diary – MS. UBC Lowry Collection 7.11.
54. C.G. McNeil in Bowker, *op. cit.*, p. 159.
55. M. Raymond, *ibid.*, p. 194.
56. *Poems*, p. 39.

Index

234

Index